# Contents

# Preface

This book examines the evidence for a relationship between organisational culture and organisational performance in the healthcare sector. It is one outcome of a larger study commissioned by the UK Department of Health. The empirical component of the study will be reported separately. Politicians, managers and others have responsibility to ensure that public sector and to a lesser extent private sector organisations are organised and managed efficiently. They are accountable for how the public's money is spent, in order to prevent waste, fraud and other inefficiencies. They are also accountable for the quality of the service that this money purchases on the public's behalf. If it is possible to analyse and intervene in any of the variables that mediate the process between expenditure and output, then these possibilities should be explored. Organisational culture has been posited as one such key 'variable'. This raises questions about whether organisational culture can be said to exist in any tangible sense, the mode of that existence, how we can gain a reliable knowledge of its existence, and how it is plausible to infer, analyse, describe or otherwise account for its existence.

The book is divided into three parts, each of which addresses an important aspect of the relationships between organisational culture and performance. Part 1 traces the development of organisational culture as a subject, surveys the different approaches to its analysis, and examines the role of leadership and the management of change. Part 2 collects all of the culture assessment tools, categorises them, and examines their application in healthcare contexts. Part 3 analyses the culture and performance link in terms of the evidence available with regard to both healthcare and non-healthcare organisations, the different scales or levels at which a relationship appears to operate, the choices to be made in deciding how to select performance assessment criteria, and how to conduct an assessment.

**Tim Scott**
*April 2003*

# Healthcare Performance and Organisational Culture

**Tim Scott**
*Research Fellow*
*Department of Health Sciences*
*University of York*
*Harkness Fellow and Visiting Scholar*
*School of Public Health*
*University of California, Berkeley*

**Russell Mannion**
*Senior Research Fellow*
*Centre for Health Economics*
*University of York*

**Huw Davies**
*Professor of Health Policy and Management*
*Department of Management*
*University of St Andrews*

**and**

**Martin Marshall**
*Professor of General Practice*
*National Primary Care Research and Development Centre*
*University of Manchester*

Radcliffe Medical Press

**Radcliffe Medical Press Ltd**
18 Marcham Road
Abingdon
Oxon OX14 1AA
United Kingdom

**www.radcliffe-oxford.com**
The Radcliffe Medical Press electronic catalogue and online ordering facility.
Direct sales to anywhere in the world.

---

British Library Cataloguing in Publication Data

A catalogue record for this book is available from the British Library.

ISBN 1 85775 914 1

Typeset by Aarontype Ltd, Easton, Bristol
Printed and bound by TJ International Ltd, Padstow, Cornwall

# About the authors

**Tim Scott** MA (Lancaster), PhD (Hull) is a Harkness Fellow in Health Care Policy, a research fellow in the Department of Health Sciences at the University of York and a visiting scholar in the Division of Health Policy and Management at the University of California, Berkeley. His research interests include organisational analysis, behaviour and symbolism, strategic change, and quality improvement in healthcare. He previously worked in the NHS Centre for Reviews and Dissemination at the University of York, and in the Centre for Health Services Studies at the University of Warwick.

**Russell Mannion** BA Hons (Stirling), PG Dip Hlth Econ (Tromso), PhD (Manchester) is a Senior Research Fellow at the Centre for Health Economics, University of York. He is also Director of the Masters course in Health Economics at the Nuffield Institute for Health, University of Leeds. His research interests embrace: performance management and measurement in healthcare; clinical governance and accountability; economic aspects of healthcare organisation and delivery; institutional economics; and international health policy reform.

**Huw TO Davies** MA (Cantab), MSc, PhD, HonMFPHM is Professor of Health Care Policy and Management at the University of St Andrews, and a former Harkness Fellow in Health Care Policy when he was based at the Institute for Health Policy Studies at the University of California, San Francisco. He is Co-Director of both the Centre for Public Policy & Management (CPPM) and the Research Unit for Research Utilisation (RURU) in the School of Social Science at St Andrews, and is Associate Director of the Pharmaco Economics Research Centre (PERC) at the same place. His research interests are in healthcare quality, encompassing evidence-based policy and practice, performance measurement and management, accountability, governance and trust. He also has a particular interest in the role of organisational culture in the delivery of high quality care.

**Martin Marshall** BSc, MB BS, MSc, MD, FRCGP is a Professor of General Practice at the National Primary Care Research and Development Centre, University of Manchester, and a part-time general practitioner in an inner-city practice. Prior to this he was a principal in general practice in Exeter for 10 years. His research interests are in the field of policy-related quality of care: the development, use and abuse of quality indicators in primary care; the public disclosure of information about performance; and the relationship between organisational culture and quality improvement. He was a Harkness Fellow in Health Care Policy in

1998-9, based at the RAND Corporation, California. He was a member of the General Medical Council/Royal College of General Practitioners working group that produced *Good Medical Practice for General Practitioners*. He is currently a member of the RCGP Research Group, an advisor to the Commission for Health Improvement and their Office for Healthcare Information, the Modernisation Agency, the National Clinical Assessment Authority, the National Patient Safety Agency and the National Primary Care Collaborative. He is vice-president of the European Working Group on Quality in Family Practice and a member of the Manchester Performance Panel.

# Acknowledgements

The authors wish to thank the UK Department of Health for funding this research. The final preparation of the manuscript was undertaken by Tim Scott while he held a Harkness Fellowship awarded by the Commonwealth Fund of New York. Thanks are also due to Kath Wright for help with the database searches, Ron Beswick, Sue Cartwright, Cary Cooper, Ron Cullen, Paula Greenwood, Sue MacKenzie, Steven Shortell, Nicholas Sieveking and Keith Stevenson for providing sample copies of their culture assessment tools, Debra Henderson for help with tracking down an elusive study, and Helen Parkinson and Jessica Hemingway for their excellent secretarial support.

*This book is dedicated to Elie, Cate, Laurie, Molly, Judith, Elizabeth, Catherine, Thomas, Bryn, Padrig and Sue, with thanks for their love and patience.*

# PART I

# A theory of organisational culture

The aim of Part 1 is to review the theoretical underpinnings to the study of what is termed 'organisational culture'. We begin by tracing the emergence of the term in the academic literature and its subsequent use in organisational analysis, behaviour and development. We then consider how a lack of consensus over the proper meaning of the term 'organisational culture' can be resolved by revising the form of the question 'What is organisational culture?'. Finally, we discuss the value of analysing healthcare organisations from an organisational culture perspective, with particular reference to the NHS.

## Introduction

It is difficult to review the topic of organisational culture succinctly. There is little agreement among scholars as to what the terms 'organisation' and 'culture' mean, how each can or should be observed or measured, or how different methodologies can be used to inform practical administration and organisational change. The difficulties are exacerbated by the rich variety of meanings that 'culture' has in everyday language. It broadly signifies a *symbolic* approach to organisations in order to study characteristic ideologies, language, dress codes, behaviour patterns, signs of status and authority, modes of deference and misbehaviour, rituals, myths and stories, prevailing beliefs, values, unspoken assumptions, etc. Some students believe that the state and development of organisations can only be managed effectively if the organisation is engaged at a symbolic level as a complex social system or subsystem of wider society. That belief is partly a response to the failure of 'classical' management theory to deliver results in terms of economy, efficiency, quality, and employee and customer satisfaction. There is also a tacit acknowledgement that occupational 'tribes' have status and rights over and above the instrumental demands of an organisation to produce goods or services.

Thus it might appear that the concept of organisational culture promises to meet both the needs of industry for greater efficiency and effectiveness, and the material and social needs of employees. Unfortunately, most approaches to organisational development offer similar promises and usually fail to deliver on one side or the other – and often on both. There are other reasons to be cautious, not least relative to organisational change and transformational narratives. Any model that is adopted to effect organisational change will have little effect on the severe objective constraints that are imposed by its environment. For example, severe and chronic staff shortages in the NHS are likely to undermine morale and reduce quality of care, irrespective of styles of leadership or the management of organisational change. Nor will such measures affect in any substantial way the demand for health services outstripping supply, or the demographic trajectory towards a higher proportion of older, sicker members of society. And these are just a few of the most obvious constraints at the macro-level. Within a health organisation's *culture* are likely to be found practices, beliefs, values and assumptions that tend by their very nature to strongly resist attempts to change them. Machiavelli was not exaggerating when he observed that: 'There is nothing more difficult to carry out, nor more doubtful of success, nor more dangerous to handle, than to initiate a new order of things' (Machiavelli, 1992). However, the opposite could equally be true – that nothing endangers an organisation more than a failure to detect a need for change and to carry the appropriate changes through, as the recent history of Marks and Spencer amply demonstrates.

We can better understand the significance of organisational culture by tracing its emergence as a distinctive approach to organisational analysis and behaviour. Although organisational culture has the trappings of a cultural anthropological approach to the study and management of organisations, and in some cases adopts explicitly anthropological methods of research (Smircich, 1983), it emerged as much from within organisation studies as from its influence by anthropology. The development of organisational culture as a subject of study can seen as a response to and to some extent an elaboration of earlier social systems and social constructionist approaches. They in turn developed as correctives to Frederick Winslow ('Speedy') Taylor's *scientific management*, the *time and motion* studies of his successor Frank B Gilbreth, and Elton Mayo's famous 'Hawthorne experiments', successively.

From at least Adam Smith's *The Wealth of Nations* (Smith, 1970) to the present day, the study of organisations has been conducted from within various different theories or paradigms (Burrell and Morgan, 1979). Organisations have been approached as if they were machines, as organisms struggling to survive in more or less competitive environments, as information and control systems (cybernetics paradigm), as political systems, as psychic prisons, as fields of flux and transformation, as instruments of domination and as cultures (Morgan, 1986). As a comprehensive review of these paradigms is beyond the scope of this report, we here offer a brief overview of developments in organisational theory and research that have contributed to the development of an organisational culture paradigm.

# A brief history of organisational culture

The term 'organisational culture' first appeared in the academic literature in an article in *Administrative Science Quarterly* (Pettigrew, 1979; Hofstede *et al.*, 1990). Its constituent themes can be traced to earlier literature on organisational analysis. Pettigrew's own empirical study of a private British boarding school appears to have been strongly influenced by Burton Clarke (Clarke, 1970). Both traced the effect of strong, idiosyncratic individuals who had founded the organisations. This concern with the role of leaders and leadership in turn highlights the influence of Selznick's *Leadership in Administration* (Selznick, 1957). Selznick distinguishes between two ideal types of enterprise – on the one hand, a rational instrumental *organisation*, and on the other, the value-infused *institution*. According to Selznick, the term 'organisation' suggests a technical instrument for harnessing human energies and directing them towards set aims, while the term 'institution' suggests an organic social entity. In the mechanistic 'organisation', tasks are allocated, authority is delegated, communications are channelled, and the whole enterprise is seen in terms of a co-ordinated rationing out of work conceived as an exercise in engineering and governed by rationality and discipline:

> The term 'organization' thus suggests a certain bareness, a lean, no-nonsense system of consciously co-ordinated activities. It refers to an *expendable tool*, a rational instrument engineered to do a job. An 'institution', on the other hand, is more nearly a product of social needs and pressures – a responsive, adaptive organism.
>
> (Selznick, 1957, p. 5)

Selznick does not suggest that any given enterprise must be either one thing or the other – although extreme cases might approach ideal organisations or institutions. Most enterprises resist easy classification, being complex mixtures of designed and responsive behaviour. Thus the formal technical system is only one side of the 'living association' that we encounter, and the formal relationships shown on an organisation chart provide a framework that is fleshed out by more spontaneous informal human behaviour: 'We see how the formal charter is given life and meaning by the informal "social constitution" in which it is embedded' (Selznick, 1957, p. 6). This institutional analysis brings attention to the emergence of 'natural' social processes within a formal association. These two aspects of an enterprise are complementary, providing a structural reference to guide individual and collective activity towards common, and sometimes uncommon, ends.

According to Selznick, the litmus test of organisation vs. institution is *expendability*. If an enterprise is a mere instrument, it can be easily cast aside. However, when an infusion of value occurs, there is resistance to change:

> People feel a sense of loss; the 'identity' of the group or community seems somehow to be violated; they bow to economic or technological considerations only reluctantly, with

regret. A case in point is the perennial effort to save San Francisco's cable cars from replacement by more economical forms of transportation. The Marine Corps has this institutional halo, and resists administrative measures that would submerge its identity.

(Selznick, 1957, p. 19)

Significantly, half a century later the institutions of San Francisco's cable cars and the US Marines still survive. However, the main topic of Selznick's analysis is *leadership*. According to Selznick, leadership is a slippery phenomenon that eludes both common sense and social science. This is partly because what leaders do is not obvious. Their leadership operates in complex and ambiguous situations that are generated by institutional life. Nor is leadership necessarily a personal trait – although it can be. Selznick's definition of leadership suggests an emergence of leaders contingent upon the types of social situations in which critical decisions are needed to influence the course of events. We shall address each of Selznick's three criteria for leadership briefly in turn.

1 *Leadership is a kind of work that is done to meet the needs of a social situation.* Selznick was influenced by the then relatively new discipline of social psychology, which viewed leadership as being contingent upon the situations in which it is observed. He supports this view by reference to post-war research, including a review of military leadership studies:

> Leadership is specific to the particular situation under investigation. Who becomes the leader of a given group engaging in a particular activity and what the leadership characteristics are in the given case are a function of the specific situation, including the measuring instruments employed*. There is a wide variation in the characteristics of individuals who become leaders in similar situations, and an even greater divergence in leadership in different situations.
>
> (Jenkins, 1947, cited in Selznick, 1957, p. 75)

Jenkins did not imagine a subpopulation of natural-born leaders in search of people to lead and projects to lead on. Who will lead, and how, depends on the context within which a need for leadership arises. Selznick does not exclude the possibility that leadership in large-scale organisations could be connected to traits of certain types of individuals. He emphasises that the specific idea of leadership with which he is concerned is a function of the dynamic social life of the institution, rather than of the static instrumental framework of the organisation. Selznick also views leaders as 'critical' decision makers who affect the strategic course of institutional activities, rather than the humdrum 'routine' decisions of everyday organisational life. He does not view leadership as infinitely variable or wholly contingent on a situation, but he invokes Stogdill's review (Stogdill, 1948) of studies of personal factors associated with leadership:

---

* We shall see later that a concern with the influence of measuring instruments on the definition of the measured object is crucial to our understanding of organisational culture.

The evidence suggests that leadership is a relation that exists between persons in a social situation, and that persons who are leaders in one situation may not necessarily be leaders in other situations. Must it then be assumed that leadership is entirely incidental, haphazard and unpredictable? Not at all. The very studies which provide the strongest arguments for the situational nature of leadership also supply the strongest evidence indicating that leadership patterns as well as non-leadership patterns of behavior are persistent and relatively stable.*

(Selznick, 1957, p. 65)

2 *Leadership is not equivalent to office holding or high prestige or authority or decision making.* Selznick's second definition follows from the previous discussion of the socially situated context of leadership. Individuals in formal positions of authority are not necessarily effective leaders. Their influence on critical as opposed to routine decision making can be minimal.

3 *Leadership is dispensable.* Leadership arises only within the dynamic, social institutional side of enterprise. The static instrumental organisation does not need leadership, according to Selznick's definition. Leadership is needed where there are critical decisions to be made. Attempts to express leadership in routine administrative situations are redundant and may be dysfunctional.

Selznick's essay has been highly influential in organisation studies. It describes the important distinction between the organisation as a rational, dispensable instrument for the production of goods or services, and as a value-infused robust social institution. Bringing people into association in the workplace, the mechanical organisation also gives birth to the dynamic social institution. Being dynamic and having a tendency to develop its own subsystemic goals, the institution requires leadership to co-ordinate its activities in relation to the instrumental means and ends of the enterprise.

These themes informed the conceptualisation and study of organisational culture, and are part of its genealogy. In common with the *human relations movement*, organisational culture emphasises the socially dynamic aspect of organisations, as against the earlier mechanistic conceptions of Taylor's *scientific management*. An infusion of the organisation by values, and an associated resistance to change, are both important aspects of the study of organisational culture. We shall examine the question of leadership and organisational culture later in this section.

Other early work on organisational analysis that is worth including in a genealogy of organisational culture is JAC Brown's *The Social Psychology of*

---

* The hypothesis of *patterns of leadership* raises questions about leadership and gender. The word 'pattern' derived from *pater* (father). The extent to which studies of leadership and organisational culture are influenced by gender issues is an important question. This is an example of how carefully we should attend to organisational language as an important dimension of culture. And this in turn should alert us to the fact that ideologies can advance behind a mask of everyday language.

*Industry* (Brown, 1954), which elaborates Roethlisberger and Dickson's (Roethlisberger and Dickson, 1939) distinction between the formal and informal organisation of the workplace. The formal organisation (to which Selznick's rational instrument organisation is similar) is the official hierarchy as it appears on an organisation chart. This traditionally consists of three main substructures, namely a line organisation (which is the formal system of authority), a functional organisation (which is based on the type of work done) and a staff structure (which is based on specialisation, e.g. engineers, designers, etc.). It was the formal organisation of the factory towards which the efficiency-improving work of Taylor and Gilbreth's *scientific management* was directed. According to Brown, the formal organisation of the workplace, so far as its theory is concerned, has three main characteristics.

1  It is deliberately impersonal.
2  It is based on ideal relationships.
3  It is based on the 'rabble' hypothesis of human nature (i.e. that workers are isolated units who may be moved about from one job to another depending entirely on their ability to do the job).

Missing from the formal theory of organisation is any recognition of the importance of workers' personalities and of their collective relationships. These relationships are defined by social or group psychologists in terms of primary and secondary groups (Sprott, 1958). Large organisations are built up from a number of smaller groups averaging about eight or ten people each. The number is limited because problems of communication increase as the size of the group increases. In the absence of adequate face-to-face communication there is a tendency for the group to break up or subdivide after it has reached a certain critical size.

Unless they are entirely independent, primary groups must communicate by setting up another executive organisation:

> That is to say, the leaders of the unit groups must not only be members of their own working units – they must join together to form an executive unit which acts as a sort of nervous system in maintaining contact between the individual groups.
>
> (Brown, 1954, p. 124)

It is this development – the primary group outgrowing its own face-to-face viability, splitting into further primary groups and thereby creating a composite whole or secondary group – which gives rise to the need for an executive function and the challenge of leadership posed by large organisations. The simultaneous contribution of an executive member to two groups and two organisational levels by a single act is a critical feature of all complex organizations. It transforms the complex into an organic whole (Barnard, 1938). When the primary groups that together form a larger organisation contribute to a common goal, that organisation is described as being well integrated.

However, if the primary groups pursue their own ends, then the organisation is described as showing a tendency towards segmentation (Brown, 1954).

According to Brown, the informal organisation of the workplace (to which Selznick's natural social institution is similar) exists at five different levels:

1  the total informal organisation of the workplace, viewed as a system of interlinked groups of all types
2  interest groups that form around 'hot' issues or internal politics. These groups may be large, diffuse, or extend through several or all departments
3  primary, face-to-face groups that are formed on the basis of shared work or location ('cliques')
4  groups of two or three intimate friends who may be part of larger cliques
5  isolated individuals who rarely participate in social activities.

The functional contribution that is made by the informal organisation to the viability of the formal organisation is crucial:

> Without the assistance of informal organization, formal organization would often be ineffective. This is frequently the case when managers try to determine every detail in production. They are too far removed from production to envisage many of the problems that arise. Yet frequently they give orders on the basis of presumed knowledge. If their orders were completely obeyed, confusion would result and production and morale would be lowered. In order to achieve the goals of the organization, workers must often violate orders, resort to their own technique of doing things, and disregard lines of authority. Without this kind of systematic sabotage, much work could not be done. This unsolicited sabotage in the form of disobedience and subterfuge is especially necessary to enable large bureaucracies to function effectively.
> (Miller and Form, *Industrial Sociology*, cited in Brown, 1954, p. 145)

Thus Brown's account of the formal and informal organisation parallels Selznick's analysis of the instrumental organisation and the value-infused institution. Both emphasise the emergence of the informal, socially organic organisation from the bare blueprint of the formal organisational structure. Both also emphasise their interdependency. Is 'organisational culture' the same as Brown's informal organisation and Selznick's institution? The problem with such a definition is that it ignores the influence of wider society on the organisation, which the analyst cannot afford to do, especially with such large, value-infused institutions as the NHS and other large health systems, including large institutions in the USA (e.g. the VA Veterans Health Administration) or Kaiser Permanente.

In fact, Brown does almost provide a definition of 'organisational culture':

> The culture of industrial groups derives from many sources: from class origins, occupational and technical sources, the atmosphere of the factory which forms their background, and, finally, from the specific experiences of the small informal group itself. Some of its more important manifestations may be classified as (a) occupational language, (b) ceremonies and rituals, and (c) myths and beliefs.
> (Brown, 1954, pp. 145–6)

An analysis of occupational language, ceremony and ritual is familiar to anyone acquainted with the literature on organisational culture. Let us therefore examine only briefly what Brown means by these terms, and sketch out their significance for analysing healthcare organisations.

# Occupational language

Technical language, including argot and jargon, is a familiar feature of occupations and institutions. Many of the terms that are used by accountants, engineers, doctors and other specialised trades are strictly technical and have no lay equivalents. In medical terminology, parts of the body, their functions and diseases have a standardised Latin nomenclature. This provides an operational and even international language which is designed to minimise ambiguity in communication. However, medical terminology also forms a symbolic boundary around the profession, showing who is in and who is out. The language used between doctors differs from that which is used between doctors and patients. The importance of occupational language and other symbols, such as white coats and stethoscopes, is highlighted by impostors who successfully pass themselves off as doctors simply by 'talking the talk' (i.e. managing the symbolic codes), sometimes for many years before they are detected. Recent NHS scandals such as the Bristol Royal Infirmary children's heart surgery tragedy (Kennedy, 2001) suggest that symbolic professional codes can even outweigh gross deficiencies in individual and collective behaviour. Like other clans, medics close ranks and protect their own.*

Although it is not mentioned by Brown, humour is another distinctive feature of the language of occupational groups. For example, a 'gallows' humour can be observed among nurses, which may help them to cope with distressing experiences. Treating disease and death humorously might shock outsiders and appear insensitive. A different interpretation is that this 'black' humour preserves sensitivity by a ritualised display of contempt for disease and suffering. 'Laughing at the devil' in this way may be a highly functional form of repression.

---

* The term 'performance' is noteworthy in this context. It is important to recognise two related senses, namely 'performance' as a dramatic reference and 'performance' as a measure of efficiency. The impostor who performs the role of doctor well may convince patients and even real medics that he or she is a real doctor. The ambiguity is compounded by the argument that even real doctors need to be able to perform the role of 'doctor' convincingly, to the satisfaction of patients and peers. Arguably, therefore, the qualified and fake doctor both practise in an ambiguous zone between the dramatic and efficient definitions of 'performance'.

# Ceremonies and rituals

All of this leads us to consider the roles of ceremony and ritual in healthcare. As Brown observes:

> All well-integrated groups, whether in the Australian Bush, the South Sea Islands or a London factory, have certain ceremonies and rituals which may be classified as *initiation rites* for the novice who is joining the firm, *rites of passage* and *rites of intensification*.
> (Brown, 1954, p. 147; our italics)

Initiation rites for the novice joining the group typically include teasing and practical joking designed to ridicule and subordinate the newcomer to the pecking order of the group — or more broadly to test his or her 'temper'. Being sent out to fetch non-existent tools, such as 'a left-handed monkey wrench', or unlikely materials, such as a tin of striped paint, are typical examples, as is coating the victim's genitals with paint or engine grease, or even worse (Ackroyd and Crowdry, 1991):

> The (mainly unconscious) function of such behaviour is to demonstrate to the newcomer his inferiority and ignorance in relation to the superiority of the group members, as a consequence of which the morale of the latter is raised simultaneously with the desire of the former to become fully initiated. The novice's attitude towards the group is tested, and his resourcefulness or lack of it made clear.
> (Brown, 1954, p. 147)

We would add that newcomers do not always accept their expected role in the established pecking order, and might successfully resist subordination attempts by demonstrating a high degree of savoir-faire.

Rites of passage are ceremonies that mark the promotion, demotion or dismissal of a group member — that is, when he or she is about to leave the group. The function of rites of passage appears to be to settle ambiguity about status and membership:

> The function of the ritual may be to manifest group identification and loyalty, to ease the process of separation from the group, to emphasize the finality of the social rupture, or merely to indicate that all past animosities are forgiven and forgotten.
> (Miller and Form, cited in Brown, 1954, p. 147)

Shaking hands, giving leaving cards, having a leaving party, gift giving and speech making are all familiar examples of rites of passage in the workplace.

Between the rites of arrival and departure are rites of intensification — that is, ceremonies which demonstrate the solidarity of the group. Rites of intensification include 'away-days', providing cakes on birthdays, wearing ritual dress, Christmas and New Year parties, sharing private jokes, and even making tea. It may be thought that these everyday activities have little connection with the complex rites and customs of pre-industrial societies, or that their significance to the smooth running of organisational life is exaggerated. Although the potlatch, the Japanese tea ceremony and the robust humour of bothy life differ widely in detail, they all function to define a group's membership and existence:

> However attenuated the form these ceremonies may take, no group worthy of the name ever assumes that membership is a mere matter of walking into it. There is no integrated or coherent social group which does not make something of a ceremony of the arrival or departure of members or take part in ceremonies which, in effect, indicate its distinctness from any other group .... There always exists the awareness of what anthropologists would call the 'in-group' and the 'out-group'.
>
> (Brown, 1954, p. 148)

# Myths, beliefs and ideologies

Myths and beliefs justify the actions of the group and explain its relationship to the wider organisation and the outside world. Strengths and weaknesses of colleagues (past and present) are exaggerated and invented to suit the theories and prejudices of the purveyor with regard to the position and status of their own group. Each occupational group (management, doctors, nurses, etc.) has its own mythology about itself and other groups. Each member is influenced by a collective mythology, as few individuals are immune to the frames of reference used by peers to make sense of a shared context. Myths are, as Brown puts it, general trends in the thought of groups, and participate in their identity and cohesion. Myths, beliefs or ideologies have a number of interesting characteristics.

1　They are functionally equivalent to wrong theories (although not necessarily wrong in every detail).
2　They are unchanged by the acquisition of correct knowledge (even extensive first-hand experience which contradicts them is unlikely to change them).
3　They influence the individual's interpretation and actions.
4　They form a more or less coherent whole which cannot be altered piecemeal.
5　The sentiments of the occupational group (e.g. management towards clinicians, or vice versa) are determined less by knowledge of the individual manager or clinician than by the sentiments which prevail in the social atmosphere which surrounds the individual. (adapted from Brown, 1954).

Thus each clinician, manager or nurse tends to be seen first as a member of a mythical class of clinicians, managers or nurses, and only later as an individual in their own right.

Both Brown's and Selznick's analyses of the rational–instrumental and social–systemic dimensions of modern organisations rest on foundations laid by the founding fathers of sociology immediately after the French Revolution.

Saint-Simon noted the rise of modern organisations and their significant role in the emerging society (Durkheim, 1958). Administrative methods, he argued, would no longer depend on physical coercion or force, nor would the administrator's authority be based upon birth or hereditary privilege. The modern administrator's authority would lead from his or her possession of 'positive' knowledge and scientific skills (Gouldner, 1959).

Saint-Simon also saw a connection between the rise of science and the professions that grew up around it, and the development of *cosmopolitanism*. He expected the new professions to be cosmopolitan in their orientation, in that practitioners' loyalties would cut across local or national organisational boundaries. This orientation towards professional values had potential both to inform and to conflict with the aims and intentions of the host organisation. This theory would predict loyalties of health professionals to be divided between a commitment to patients and an allegiance to their professional group.

Saint-Simon's disciple, Auguste Compte, was less sensitive to the significance of planned organisation in the emerging society, believing its utility to be limited to dealing with serious threats to society in order to preserve its integrity. Compte was convinced that the 'final order which arises spontaneously is always superior to that which human combination had, by anticipation, constructed'.* According to Compte, therefore, the natural and spontaneous emergence and maintenance of social order are counterposed to planned, rational, political, legal organisation (Gouldner, 1959).

The distinctive rational–legal features of modern organisation were not systematically explored until Max Weber's work on bureaucracy. Like Saint-Simon, Weber saw bureaucracy as a necessary alternative to heredity, privilege, ad hoc administration and reward by grace and favour. He also saw more clearly than Saint-Simon that authority in bureaucracy could not rest on science and technology alone. Weber regarded bureaucracy as Janus faced. He saw that it was on the one side a form of administration based on knowledge and expertise, but also that authority in the modern organisation was, in some measure, always dependent upon non-rational elements (Gouldner, 1959).

Although by 'non-rational elements' Weber chiefly meant authority incumbent on office, we can extend his meaning to refer to what JAC Brown elaborates as the informal organisation and to Selznick's value-infused institution. Thus even during the early development of organisational analysis we find two distinct models of modern, large-scale organisation, namely a rational model, exemplified by Weber's work on bureaucracy,† and a natural-system model, derived from Compte, exemplified by Talcott Parsons and worked over by many later scholars. The rational model implies a mechanistic conception of

---

*Compte A (1911) *Early Essays on Social Philosophy* (translated by HD Hutton). George Routledge and Sons, London, p. 325, cited in Gouldner, 1959, p. 401.
† Weber is often misrepresented as advocating the bureaucratic form of modern organisation.

organisation as a structure, each part of which is separately modifiable with a view to enhancing the efficiency of the whole:

> Individual organizational elements are seen as subject to successful and planned modification, enactable by deliberate decision. The long-range development of the organization as a whole is also regarded as subject to planned control and as capable of being brought into increasing conformity with explicitly held plans and goals.
>
> (Gouldner, 1959, p. 405)

The natural-system model conceives the organisation holistically and views the realisation of rational organisational goals as only one of several functions to which the organisation contributes. According to this model, the organisation strives to maintain its equilibrium or survival, which may sometimes lead to the neglect or distortion of more formal organisational goals:

> Whatever the plans of their creators, organizations, say the natural-system theorists, become ends in themselves and possess their own distinctive needs which have to be satisfied. Once established, organizations tend to generate new ends which constrain subsequent decisions and limit the manner in which the nominal group goals can be pursued.
>
> (Gouldner, 1959, p. 405)

The natural-system model is based on an underlying organismic metaphor, and draws attention to the interdependence of the component parts. Planned changes are expected to have consequences, often unintended, for the entire system. Thus natural-system theorists view the organisation as having a 'life' of its own, a distinctive 'natural history' in relation to which formal interventions to modify parts or all of the system are viewed as disruptive of the system's natural evolution, perhaps leading to catastrophic consequences.

The basic polarity between rational instrumental and natural-system models of organisation has provided a theoretical context within which much organisational thinking, writing and practice have developed. The perceived challenge of reconciling these two conceptions of organisation has also received ample attention. The concept of an organisational culture can be seen fundamentally as a development of the natural-system concept, of Selznick's institution and of Brown's informal organisation.

Thus although the term 'organisational culture' may have been introduced to the literature by Pettigrew as late as 1979, it is nonetheless rooted in the work of Brown, Selznick and others (e.g. Barnard, Gouldner and Saint-Simon), who perceived the cultural aspects of organisational life and the need to incorporate their analysis into the study and management of organisations. This genealogy is evidence that a cultural approach to organisational analysis is more than a mere fad. Its recognition and refinement since the 1940s have been steady and sustained. Indeed, so long as we have groups of people associated in common enterprise, it is difficult to see how a concept of organisational culture could become redundant.

# How has organisational culture been analysed?

A number of scholars have surveyed the literature on organisational culture that has appeared since the late 1970s (Smircich, 1983; Allaire and Firsirotu, 1984; Meek, 1988; Ott, 1989; Schein, 1990; Brown, 1995; Parker, 2000). Each imposes a different organising framework on to this large and diverse field. Our modest aim here is to present a brief account, focusing on aspects that are relevant to the study of health organisational cultures.

The absence of an intrinsic structure to organisational culture studies reflects the idea that culture is an emergent property, like improvised theatre. (Whether any deeper pattern or structure exists that is common to all organisational cultures is too complex a debate to address here.) As players in such a performance, we lack precise scripts. Our rehearsals are our previous performances in other situations. 'Critics' (researchers, reviewers and other writers) report their perceptions about the 'plot' and 'performance', but these are different from the perceptions of the 'players'. The performance is a co-operative enterprise, and later on we shall consider the ways in which and extent to which leaders may write, produce and direct the organisational cultural production. The leader is just another player cast in the important role of 'leader'.

The dramatic perspective outlined in the previous paragraph is an example of an organisational 'paradigm', 'metaphor' or 'image' (Morgan, 1986). It enables us to view organisational culture from a specific 'perspective' (orientation metaphor) or through a particular 'lens' (optical metaphor). This simple but powerful technique allows us to generate different perceptions and assessments of situations according to the paradigm selected. Taking the argument a stage further, approaching organisational culture using metaphors allows us to generate a plurality of organisations, not merely different views of the 'same' organisation. We cannot avoid metaphors (the term 'organisation' is itself a metaphor), as they are an essential building block of thought and language. Organisational *culture* is an anthropological metaphor. The lack of consensus over the meaning of the term 'culture' in anthropology is matched by the variety of its applications to organisational analysis and development. We could laboriously excavate fragments of organisational culture from the mountains of literature, and hope that by piecing them carefully together a whole skeleton would be assembled (archaeological/forensic metaphor). However, that undertaking is beyond the scope of this book, and in any case is probably misguided. Archaeology, like history, is always partial, always based on a sample of the available artefacts, which are a minute sample of the culture that produced them and therefore unrepresentative of a whole, which probably never existed in any case. The skeleton is a montage of bits and pieces belonging to different bodies – even different species – from different periods. Our aim here is to examine what it means to study organisations as cultures, including a brief consideration of appropriate research methodologies. We argued above that organisational culture is more than a fad in the management and academic literature. Its main constituent themes of organisational symbolism, rites and rituals, myths and ideologies, and leadership have been worked over and refined since the 1950s. However, a popular interest in organisational culture developed in the 1980s after attempts to explain why US companies had fallen behind those in other countries, notably Japan, in terms of quality control, competitiveness and expansion. It was thought that the answer lay in being able to differentiate, analyse and manipulate organisational cultures (Ouchi, 1981; Pascale and Athos, 1981; Schein, 1990). It was thought that by actively managing an organisation's culture, it should be possible to transplant the cultural strengths of a Toyota or a Mitsubishi into a General Motors, creating cultural hybrids that Ouchi termed 'Z' companies. Lacking any robust *evidence* to support theory, an ideology of organisational culture sprang up, fuelled by Peters and Waterman's bestseller *In Search of Excellence* (Peters and Waterman, 1982) and the glut of pulp management fiction on the subject that followed. Serious students of organisation became interested in the phenomenon and began to explore the implications of what it really meant to study organisations as if they were cultures.

In an elegant article, Smircich has analysed how culture has emerged in organisation studies through two perspectives – as a critical variable and as a 'root' metaphor (Smircich, 1983). Her analysis demonstrates that organisational analysts have held varying conceptions of culture, giving rise to different research questions and interests and different research agendas. A summary of Smircich's paper will help to define what it can mean to study health organisations as cultures, drawing from different approaches to organisation theory and social anthropology.

We have noted how organisational analysts and managers tend to utilise a variety of metaphors or images (Morgan, 1980, 1986) to generate insights into organisational life. The metaphors of machine and organism have been most pervasive (Pondy and Mitroff, 1979; Morgan, 1980; Koch and Deetz, 1981; Morgan, 1986), such that the ideas and terms generated by them have become incorporated into common language, whereas their metaphorical influence continues largely unnoticed. In this manner, theories decay into assumptions. Several authors have analysed the range of assumptions that organisation theorists bring to their subject (Ritzer, 1975; Burrell and Morgan, 1979; Morgan and Smircich, 1980; Van de Ven and Astley, 1981; Ott, 1989). There is general agreement that the field of organisation theory can be characterised by a range of assumptions located on an objective–subjective continuum about reality and how we can know it, and a range of assumptions on the determinist–voluntarist question about human nature and society. It has been argued that the metaphorical process of seeing one thing in terms of another is a fundamental element of thought and how we make sense of the world (Lackoff and Johnson, 1980). There is also a general belief that organisations are highly resistant to

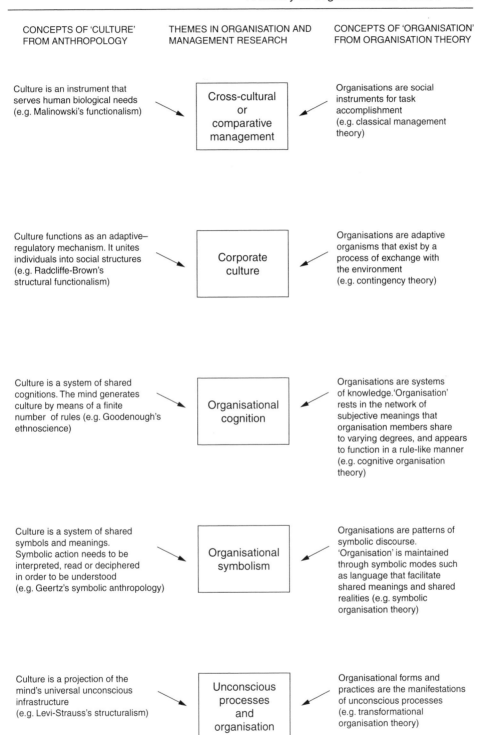

CONCEPTS OF 'CULTURE'
FROM ANTHROPOLOGY

THEMES IN ORGANISATION AND
MANAGEMENT RESEARCH

CONCEPTS OF 'ORGANISATION'
FROM ORGANISATION THEORY

Culture is an instrument that
serves human biological needs
(e.g. Malinowski's functionalism)

Cross-cultural
or
comparative
management

Organisations are social
instruments for task
accomplishment
(e.g. classical management
theory)

Culture functions as an adaptive–
regulatory mechanism. It unites
individuals into social structures
(e.g. Radcliffe-Brown's
structural functionalism)

Corporate
culture

Organisations are adaptive
organisms that exist by a
process of exchange with
the environment
(e.g. contingency theory)

Culture is a system of shared
cognitions. The mind generates
culture by means of a finite
number of rules (e.g. Goodenough's
ethnoscience)

Organisational
cognition

Organisations are systems
of knowledge. 'Organisation'
rests in the network of
subjective meanings that
organisation members share
to varying degrees, and appears
to function in a rule-like manner
(e.g. cognitive organisation
theory)

Culture is a system of shared
symbols and meanings.
Symbolic action needs to be
interpreted, read or deciphered
in order to be understood
(e.g. Geertz's symbolic anthropology)

Organisational
symbolism

Organisations are patterns of
symbolic discourse.
'Organisation' is maintained
through symbolic modes such
as language that facilitate
shared meanings and shared
realities (e.g. symbolic
organisation theory)

Culture is a projection of the
mind's universal unconscious
infrastructure
(e.g. Levi-Strauss's structuralism)

Unconscious
processes
and
organisation

Organisational forms and
practices are the manifestations
of unconscious processes
(e.g. transformational
organisation theory)

**Figure 1.1**  Intersections of culture and organisation theory (adapted from Smircich, 1983).

analysis, and even more recalcitrant to change. Thus the ethic has grown in the field that organisations do not respond well to head-on confrontations, and that subtler analytical approaches are likely to meet with more success. It follows from this logic that metaphors have tended to compensate for the weaknesses of their predecessors. Thus the conception of an organisation running like a well-oiled machine, or breaking down and needing mechanical repair, was ultimately seen to lack much understanding of an organisation as a social system. The conception of an organisation as an organism struggling for survival within a determinate environment compensated for that weakness by focusing on inter-actions between organisational socio-technical subsystems and the surrounding social, commercial, political and technical systems (Trist and Bamforth, 1951; Burns and Stalker, 1961; Lawrence and Lorsch, 1967). The conception of an organisation as culture takes the social systems perspective a stage further to include an examination of the symbolic aspects of social organisation, which was previously lacking.

Smircich (1983) has identified five different programmes of research into organisational cultures (*see* Figure 1.1). Each programme emerges at the inter-section of matching anthropological and organisational concepts.

# Culture and comparative management: culture as an independent variable

Comparative management assesses managerial and employee practices across countries (Haire *et al.*, 1966). From this perspective, culture is considered to be synonymous with nationality. There are two main streams of research into comparative management, namely a macro focus examining the relationships between culture and organisational structure and functioning, and a micro focus examining the similarities and differences in managerial attitudes between cultures (Everett *et al.*, 1982). The literature is extensive, but perhaps the most famous work is Ouchi's *Theory Z* (Ouchi, 1981), which is a comparison between US and Japanese industrial cultures.

The practical utility of comparative management is relevant to multinational organisations (Hofstede, 1980; Hofstede *et al.*, 1990) and international trade. Cross-cultural management studies may be useful to international studies of health organisational culture. Intra-national studies on the dimension of ethnic subculture may also be useful as some health organisational cultures, such as those in the UK and the USA, emerge in part through interaction between the members of different ethnic groups (both practitioners and patients) with different health expectations, attitudes, assumptions and practices.

# Corporate culture: culture as an internal variable

Organisations are culture producing as well as culture consuming (Louis, 1980; Deal and Kennedy, 1982; Martin and Powers, 1983; Schein, 1985, 1990, 1999). In Selznick's terms (Selznick, 1957), the instrumental organisation of enterprise brings people together in association, which then produces a value-infused institution. Corporate culture studies address the value-infused institution complete with its artefacts, such as symbolic codes of behaviour, rituals (Deal and Kennedy, 1982), myths (Boje *et al.*, 1982), ideologies (Harrison, 1972), stories (Mitroff and Kilmann, 1976), legends (Wilkins and Martin, 1980) and specialised language (Andrews and Hirsch, 1983).

According to this model, culture is defined as the social or normative glue that holds an organisation together (Siehl and Martin, 1981; Tichy, 1982). Several authors have argued that 'strong' cultures are more successful than 'weak' ones (Deal and Kennedy, 1982; Peters and Waterman, 1982). However, the evidence for this assertion is poor. Several of the companies cited by Peters and Waterman (1982) as paragons of excellence later fell on hard times. One has only to consider examples such as Marks and Spencer, British Rail and the NHS to locate organisations with very strong cultures that have apparently offered no particular or reliable commercial advantages. Moreover, the shrinkage of traditional fee-for-service health insurance and the rise of health maintenance organisations in the USA had little to do with organisational culture and a great deal to do with market forces.

The concept of corporate culture as an internal variable has been closely associated with *organisational development* (OD) (Jacques, 1952; Harrison, 1972; Schein, 1990). Practitioners of OD tend to adopt a 'clinical' perspective (Schein, 1985), helping organisations to make strategically important decisions and overcome problems that require an outsider's viewpoint. OD interventions are often directed at the organisational culture, and aim to question the espoused values and underlying assumptions under which employees operate (French and Bell, 1978; Schein, 1985, 1990, 1999).

> These activities then serve to make the culture more receptive to change, facilitating the realignment of the total organizational system into a more viable and satisfying configuration.
>
> (Smircich, 1983, p. 345)

Other corporate culture research has been less focused on planned organisational change, but has still been concerned with the effects of various dimensions of organisational culture on a variety of outcomes, including the function of managerial ideologies and organisational stories in hospitals (Meyer, 1981), the symbolic power of information (Martin and Powers, 1983), and management as symbolic action (Pfeffer, 1981). These authors share a basic view that cultural artefacts, including management styles, are powerful symbolic means of communication:

> They can be used to build organizational commitment, convey a philosophy of management, rationalize and legitimate activity, motivate personnel, and facilitate socialization.
> (Smircich, 1983, p. 345)

The corporate culture that is conceived as comprising shared key values and beliefs fulfils several important functions (*see* Box 1.1).

---

**Box 1.1**   Functions of corporate culture (adapted from Smircich, 1983)

1 It conveys a sense of identity for organisation members.
2 It facilitates commitment to something larger than the self.
3 It enhances social systems stability.
4 It provides a sense-making device to guide behaviour.

---

Corporate culture conveys a sense of identity for organisation members (Deal and Kennedy, 1982; Peters and Waterman, 1982). It involves commitment to an entity larger than the self (Siehl and Martin, 1981; Peters and Waterman, 1982), it moderates social system stability (Louis, 1980), and culture provides a sense-making device or context to guide and shape behaviour (Louis, 1980; Meyer, 1981; Pfeffer, 1981; Siehl and Martin, 1981). However, the key question for corporate culture theorists is whether corporate culture as an internal variable can be manipulated to influence the *performance* of the organisation. The research agenda arising from this perspective focuses on how to change an organisation's culture in order to bring it in line with management's purposes. Its weakness lies in the exclusivity of this focus. In talking about *an* organisational culture, one loses sight of the great likelihood that there are multiple organisational subcultures, and indeed countercultures, competing to define the nature of situations. Messianic appeals to take managerial control of the corporate culture tend to be over-optimistic and destined to disappoint managers who may be willing to grasp at any straw to stop themselves drowning in the organisational chaos that appears to confront them. We must therefore question whether corporate culture is more than just another ideology of control. If it is, it is impressive in its ambition not merely to oil the wheels of industry, but to redefine the organisational reality *per se*, to legitimate one view of organisational life and suppress others by covertly manipulating overt cultural symbols.* This is a totalising image of hegemony – of managers attempting to control the bodies of employees by acquiring the keys to their minds and perhaps even their souls.

---

* This is also the definition of propaganda (JAC Brown, 1963).

# Culture as a variable: summary

Comparative management and corporate culture are both consistent with the functionalist paradigm (Burrell and Morgan, 1979). Both assume that the social world can be defined in terms of distinct, interacting variables (Morgan and Smircich, 1980). This is a variant of the organismic metaphor of organisation as a living subsystem that is struggling for survival in an environment that presents imperative stimuli (usually termed 'information') to behaviour. Comparative management regards culture as part of the environment which exerts a patterning or imprinting influence on the organisation. Corporate culture views culture as a product of human enactment. Underlying both approaches is a search for predictable methods for organisational control.

# Culture as a root metaphor

The comparative and corporate perspectives outlined above view culture as something that an organisation has – either by dint of its location within a wider social system, or through its indigenous generation of institutional symbols, norms and values. Other theorists take a more radical view – that culture is something that an organisation *is* (Smircich, 1983). This marks a shift in focus from culture as a distinctive variable to culture as the context of all organisational variables. To state that this means a shift to researching organisations from an anthropological perspective rather than a consultant one is inadequate, as anthropologists are not an homogeneous group, any more than organisational analysts are. Smircich defines three ways of approaching organisations *as* cultures (*see* Figure 1.1) – through a cognitive perspective, through a symbolic perspective, and through structural and psychodynamic perspectives (Smircich, 1983).

# Cognitive perspective

Culture has been studied as a system of shared ideas (Goodenough, 1971), knowledge or beliefs (Rossi and O'Higgins, 1980). For example, Harris and Cronin (1979) view an organisational culture as a particular structure of knowledge that informs understanding and action. They term this structure a 'master contract' that includes the organisation's self-image and a set of rules that organise beliefs and behaviour in the light of that image. The master contract develops out of interpersonal interaction and provides the context for further interaction. Harris and Cronin's methodology examines the contract/self-image and the degree of consensus on its constructs, and assesses co-orientation (the extent to which members perceive others' construction of the organisational image accurately) and co-ordination (the extent to which members can organise their knowledge of the organisational image into rules for functional, co-operative action).

Other researchers who have used a cognitive approach to organisational culture include Argyris and Schon (1978), Bougon (1983), Wacker (1981) and Weick (1979a, 1979b). Argyris and Schon (1978) have used use a case-building approach to examine members' 'theories in use' to guide their interaction. They distinguish between single-loop and double-loop learning. Single-loop learning relates to feedback on actions limited to the existing theory in use, whereas double-loop learning refers to a more radical learning that involves a shift in the theory in use.

## Symbolic perspective

A number of authors have called attention to the power of organisational symbolism, legends, stories, myths and ceremonies (Brown, 1954; Mitroff and Kilmann, 1976; Martin and Powers, 1983; Morgan *et al.*, 1983; Trice and Beyer, 1984). From this perspective, an organisational culture is interpreted as symbolic discourse. Any organisational artefact can (and indeed must) have a symbolic significance. The physical layout of the workplace symbolises relationships. A spacious office symbolises the status of an executive in a similar way to that in which a row of racks and benches symbolises IT staff, or an open-plan design symbolises teamwork. An organisation's products or services are also symbolic both to the staff who produce and deliver them and to the customers and clients who consume them. Health organisations are loaded with symbolism, including uniforms (e.g. white coats, theatre scrubs, suits) and accessories (e.g. stethoscopes, prescription pads), waiting-rooms (possibly symbolising a subordination of patients to the system), wards (symbolising supervision, order and control), and so on.

We cannot adequately interpret these material artefacts in isolation from the values and assumptions of the organisation. For example, an open-plan office design might suggest a democratic workplace, but it might just as easily constitute a dysfunctional design in relation to values of individual expertise and a need for privacy in order to do meticulous or confidential work. We cannot therefore take symbolic artefacts at face value. Usually they form a code which the organisational analyst decodes, interprets, 'reads' (Turner, 1983) or 'deciphers' (Van Maanen, 1973). The focus of such an analysis is the way in which participants themselves make sense of their experience and how that relates to their behaviour. This focus of interest is shared by symbolic organisation theorists and organisational leaders. Both are concerned with how a sense of organisation is created and maintained, and how to achieve common inter-pretations of situations and events so that co-ordinated action is possible. Some authors argue explicitly that leadership should be understood as the management of meaning and the shaping of interpretations (Peters, 1978; Smircich and Morgan, 1982).

It might appear that organisational symbolists are concerned with a some-what peripheral and nebulous dimension of organisational life. However, from the perspective of symbolic anthropology, symbolic discourse suffuses cultural and organisational life so completely that no separation between non-symbolic 'things' and symbolic codes is possible. If one considers the range of symbolic interpretations of an everyday object such as a disposable syringe, the difficulty of this separation becomes very clear. The syringe symbolises medicine and pain, effective drug administration and needlestick injury, sterility and risk of cross-infection, drug abuse, HIV/AIDS, disposability and dangerous waste, etc. The syringe *is* all of these things and *has* all of these meanings simul-taneously. That is what makes it an ambiguous and potent symbol.

## Structural and psychodynamic perspectives

Culture can also be interpreted as the expression of unconscious psychological and psychodynamic processes (Yiannis, 1999). This perspective adopts a Freu-dian approach to the interpretation of organisational culture as a relationship between latent unconscious and manifest conscious levels. From this perspective:

> Organisational forms and practices are understood as projections of unconscious processes and are analysed with reference to the dynamic interplay between out-of-awareness processes and their conscious manifestation.
>
> (Smircich, 1983, p. 351)

One example of this approach is Turner's application of a structural anthropo-logical analysis (after Levi-Strauss) in order to understand differences between bureaucratic and industrial forms of organisation, and to diagnose organisa-tional conflicts (Turner, 1977, 1983). Another example is Mitroff's application of Jungian cultural archetypes to investigate structural patterns linking the unconscious human mind with its manifestations in social organisation (Mitroff, 1982). These approaches turn on a belief in a deep underlying structure of mind, of which human culture and organisation are manifest expressions. Their key significance to researching organisational culture is that what is perceived at the surface of organisational life becomes adequately meaningful only as an expression of the deep underlying forces of the unconscious.

## *Culture as a root metaphor: summary*

By adopting culture as a root metaphor, cognitive, symbolic, structuralist and psychodynamic theorists all share a view of organisation as a particular form of human individual and social expression. This is a very different approach to viewing the organisation as a machine or an adaptive organism. Instead of viewing language, symbols, myths, stories and rituals as cultural artefacts, as in the culture-as-variable approach, the root metaphor interprets these phenomena as generative processes that are intrinsic to a culture and to organisational life:

> When culture is a root metaphor, the researcher's attention shifts from concerns about what do organizations accomplish and how may they accomplish it more efficiently, to how is organization accomplished and what does it mean to be organized?
>
> (Smircich, 1983, p. 353)

Pettigrew (1979) and Pondy and Mitroff (1979) advocated that organisation theory should move beyond open-system models of organisation to a cultural model. As we have seen, the key themes of such an approach were described earlier by JAC Brown (Brown, 1954), including a concern with occupational language, symbols, myths and ideologies. The approaches summarised above show how the concepts of organisation and culture have been linked, and their accompanying research agendas. What unites all of these approaches to organisation is the focus on the expressive, non-rational, subjective and interpretive dimensions of organisational life.

# Organisational subcultures

One aspect of organisational culture that was first raised by Saint-Simon concerns the emergence of cosmopolitanism among professions, whose loyalties cut across organisational boundaries (Gouldner, 1959). The significance of professional identity and orientation may be one key to help unlock the culture of healthcare organisations. Most reviews of organisational culture start by asking the question 'What is organisational culture?'. This is fundamentally the wrong form of question. We should in fact ask '*Which* organisational culture?'. The NHS, for example, is a distinctively British institution that is influenced by British culture. It has a recognisable, unified identity and espouses certain core values. Although these factors imply an overall organisational culture, the NHS also contains organisational subcultures whose relationship to the overall organisational culture is difficult to decipher and explain. These subcultures can be categorised as shown in Box 1.2.

If a health organisation culture is a complex of subcultures, its analysis involves an assessment of the specific subcultural mix that obtains overall, or in

---

**Box 1.2**   NHS organisational subcultures

Ethnic
Religious
Class
Occupational
Divisional/specialist
Technical
Gender
Primary group
Secondary group

---

any particular location, depending on the focus. This applies to those sub-cultural influences that both providers and patients bring to the situation. From the outset, therefore, any analysis of a health organisational culture faces the following difficulty. How can the overall culture be described or assessed when it is composed of an amalgam of different subcultural strands, each of which is likely to vary from one location to another? One answer is that the analysis should reflect the scale on which it is conducted. Thus an assessment of the *overall* NHS culture, for instance, is unlikely to contain the same level of detail that a more localised study could convey. This list of subcultural influences is intended to alert the investigator to some of the potentially important influences that might need to be considered by an analysis of NHS organisational culture. The list is not intended to be exhaustive, or to indicate the relative importance of the different subcultural influences.


# Ethnic subculture

A significant proportion of practitioners and patients in UK and US healthcare organisations are members of so-called minority ethnic groups,* and may bring distinctive values and expectations about health and healthcare to the scene.†

---

*The hierarchy that is implied by culture and subculture is not intended to subordinate any subcultural dimensions absolutely, still less to imply disrespect for any ethnic culture. The terminology is merely intended to signify their relative influence on the construction and maintenance of an organisational culture.

† Hofstede G (1980) *Culture's Consequences: international differences in work-related values.* Sage, Beverly Hills, CA. Hofstede G and Bond MH (1988) The Confucius connection: from cultural roots to economic growth. *Organiz Dynamics.* **16**: 4–21. Both of these references argue that differences in national/ethnic cultures offer important clues to understanding organisational cultures.

These influences may lead to a different emphasis in the care that is delivered by different teams or individual staff to different patients, and to different expectations on the part of patients. A distinction between culture and sub-culture is complicated by the phenomenon whereby representatives of one or more ethnic groups may represent the majority of the population that is served by the healthcare organisation under study.

# Religious subculture

Differing religious beliefs can also affect preferences with regard to the types of healthcare that are offered and received. For example, Catholics believe strongly in the sanctity of the life of an unborn foetus, whereas Jehovah's Witnesses do not believe in accepting blood transfusions.*

# Class subculture

Social class has long been recognised as a determinant of occupational culture (Brown, 1954). The link between entry into professions such as medicine and the middle class is well recognised. This could be important in view of the new emphasis on concordance in decision making between doctor and patient, and correct treatment prescribing and patient compliance with a treatment plan. The success of the medical encounter is heavily dependent on successful communication between practitioner and patient. This may not occur if basic differences stemming partly from class exist and remain unexplored.

# Occupational subculture

Although they are closely associated in the common enterprise of delivering healthcare, managers, physicians, nurses, therapists, clerks, porters, cleaners and other occupational groups each have a distinctive sense of identity and

---

* A case is reported in the *British Medical Journal* of a surgeon who, being a Jehovah's Witness, practised 'bloodless' surgery. Such examples of counterculture are potentially important. If one surgeon can successfully perform surgery without blood infusions, why is it that others cannot or do not? The practice of bloodless surgery challenges a fundamental assumption of modern surgery – that the patient will inevitably bleed profusely and need to have this blood replaced. Is blood transfusion in surgery always necessary or is it related to a *surgical subculture?*

purpose. This arises from their specialised training and education, daily practice of work and interaction with peers and other occupational groups, and the attitudes, beliefs and assumptions that are thus engendered. One characteristic of the NHS is the robustness of each occupational culture and the minimal degree of cross-subcultural learning. Members of occupational groups in the NHS are indeed cosmopolitan in that their distinctive approaches to patient care are probably influenced more by the techniques, values and assumptions of their specific occupational group than by the aims and objectives of the health-care organisation to which they belong. Their orientation is professional more than corporate.

Thus a key characteristic of healthcare organisations is the range of distinc-tive and vivid occupational subcultures which provide the 'raw' material for its organisational culture. Except that the material is not raw, it is always already 'cooked' or prefabricated. Medical and nursing subcultures are cohesive, robust and resistant to change. They do not intermingle much, but rather they form distinct subcultural strata (providing a ready-made hierarchy) from which the organisation's character forms and evolves. One could imagine the stratifica-tion and deformation over time of geological forms, where each layer contacts other layers only along the fine borderline where one stratum ends and the next one begins. Studies of the interactions between doctors and nurses tend to support this idea – doctors talk mostly to other doctors of a similar rank, and the same is true of nurses. The corollary of this metaphor might be that as a subcultural laminate, NHS organisational culture would be seen to be very strong and integrated, but also highly resistant to change or deformation. The culture glue which binds them so firmly together also keeps them apart, the integrity of the whole depending on the integrity of the parts. By their very nature, subcultures do not easily 'bleed into' one another.

Another implication of an occupational subculture analysis is that the occu-pational subcultures transcend any single NHS organisation because they infuse the entire NHS culture. They also transcend individuals within the organisa-tion, subordinating attitudes and behaviour to constantly reinforced norms. This might help to explain both the scandalous behaviour of some groups, and the rarity of 'whistle blowing' to expose that behaviour. In this sense, therefore, occupational subcultures are one of the great strengths of healthcare organisations, but they are also a potential weakness because of their tendency to ignore the aims of a pan-organisational culture.

Particular healthcare organisations (hospitals, practices, etc.) can be regarded as conjunctions in the network of occupational and other subcultures. It could be postulated that each health organisation is a unique cultural configuration because the subcultures that traverse the organisational culture interact and cohere differently, reflecting individual and group characteristics and the local environment. How then can organisations that have strong common attributes (their occupational subcultures), but which are also different, be compared? One way would be to assess the relative strengths and character of the occupational subcultures that are in play within specific organisational contexts, in terms of their relationships, functioning and dysfunctioning.

# Divisional/specialist subculture

Occupational groups comprising healthcare organisations are generally sub-divided into specialisms and services (cardiology, oncology, gynaecology and obstetrics, etc.). Overlaid on the basic occupational culture, therefore, we might expect each specialism to elaborate its own distinctive subculture, based on the anatomical functions, diseases, complications, procedures and therapies that it deals with.

# Technical subculture

Related to occupation and specialism are the distinctive technologies that are utilised for examination, diagnosis and treatment. A classical investigation that involves these and other subcultural influences is presented by Joan Emmerson in her account of how participants sustain definitions of reality in gynaecological examinations (Emmerson, 1973). What is so interesting about this account is how the participants cope with the threatening situation in which the patient needs to expose her genitals for examination in a semi-public setting. Emmerson approaches the analysis from a dramaturgical perspective. The woman, especially if she is unused to the situation, is uncertain how to act appropriately (e.g. whether some display of modesty is in order). The physician adheres to a medical definition of the situation by adopting a matter-of-fact attitude. The nurse, whose main task is to act as chaperone, 'has in mind a typology of responses patients have to this situation, and a typology of doctors' styles of performance' (Emmerson, 1973, p. 360). What is striking about these responses is that they are performed or acted out with the specific purpose of defining the *normality* of the situation. In so doing they simultaneously high-light the very *abnormality* of the situation that calls for the performance:

> Although most people realise that sexual responses are inappropriate, they may be unable to dismiss the sexual reaction privately and it may interfere with the conviction with which they undertake their impersonal performance. The structure of the gynaeco-logical examination highlights the very features which the participants are supposed to dis-attend. So the more attentive the participants are to the social situation, the more the unmentionable is forced on their attention.
>
> (Emmerson 1973, p. 360)

Emmerson's study is a rare example of a focused anthropological analysis of a particular type of health encounter. Similar investigations of the influence of different medical technologies would undoubtedly yield important information about health system cultures and subcultures. Much research has been conducted on the medical encounter, particularly at the primary care level. Much of that research in turn has treated the consulting room as an extension of the laboratory, limiting the analysis to counting responses in which only some psychologists and sociologists are interested. Expanding the purview of this area of research to include aspects of healthcare organisational culture, as enacted both by patients and by practitioners, would advance our understanding of the behaviour of both practitioners and patients. One may imagine how much information could be discovered by studies similar to that of Emmerson of surgical teams, intensive-care units, oncology treatments, imaging techniques, etc. Such studies have the potential to provide new and concrete opportunities to describe and assess organisational cultures in action.

# Gender subculture

It is no longer fashionable to deny differences between the sexes. Serious students in this area are more concerned to explore the differences which identification with one gender or the other confers (Calas and Smircich, 1996). The likelihood that masculine and feminine subcultures exist within NHS organisational culture is partly related to an unequal distribution of the sexes within and between the main occupational groups. That the medical profession is dominated by men hardly needs stating. It is generally acknowledged that women suffer severe disadvantages when competing with men for the top jobs. However, our point here is less to do with equality or equity than with whatever distinctively masculine and feminine approaches to healthcare delivery and consumption men and women bring to the organisational culture. On the side of the practitioner, men might be expected to be more rational and objective and less sympathetic than female practitioners. Whether these caricatures have any foundation either in society or in healthcare is an empirical question. Admitting for the moment the possibility that they have some validity, two further speculations may be added. First, if the dominant values and assumptions held by a particular occupation are 'masculine' or feminine', it might be expected that those who are highly successful in that occupation would generally need to have internalised its dominant values, irrespective of their sex. Thus if medicine is male dominated, we would postulate that masculine values and assumptions would inform the behaviour of both men and women in that profession. Similarly, if nursing is dominated by feminine values and assumptions, then we would postulate that successful male nurses would have internalised these feminine values.

The second speculation concerns the hierarchical relationship between the professions. It is plausible that the dominant values and assumptions of the medical profession, for example, tend to inform other healthcare professions, such that a masculine hegemony exists throughout the health system. If this is so, it is possible that those who are most successful in a subordinate profession, such as nursing, are so because they have adopted the values and assumptions of the dominant medical profession. In this case these individuals would not be exemplars of their own occupational culture, but aspirants to the dominant occupational culture.

We make no truth claims for the foregoing discussion. Our aim is simply to highlight how associations of men and women in unequal numbers in different occupations might influence the organisational culture. Moreover, the identity and espoused values of the professions are vulnerable to constant social reconstruction, as Fox (1993) argues. In this and other subcultural influences the most important message is *not* to make assumptions about an organisational culture, but rather to investigate the influence of such subcultures as seem likely to exist within the organisation.

We need to look at gender subculture from the patient's perspective, too. The contribution of patients as well as practitioners to the construction and evolution of healthcare organisational culture has not been adequately recognised or addressed in the literature. It is possible that practitioners may respond differently to male and female patients. There are some obvious prompts to do this. As Emmerson (1973) observed, signs of sexual interest between health practitioners and patients are taboo, and social competencies are required to define unaccustomed behaviour in semi-public settings.

## Primary group subculture

The basic social unit of organisational analysis is the primary group. A primary group is composed of up to about 12 individuals who have regular face-to-face contact with one another. The term 'primary group' was coined by Charles Cooley:

> By primary groups I mean those characterized by intimate face-to-face association and co-operation. They are primary in several senses, but chiefly in that they are fundamental in forming the social nature and ideals of the individual. The result of intimate association ... is a certain fusion of individualities in a common whole, so that one's very self, for many purposes at least, is the common life and purpose of the group. Perhaps the simplest way of describing this wholeness is by saying that it is a 'we'; it involves the sort of sympathy and mutual identification for which 'we' is the natural expression.
>
> (Cooley, 1909, p. 23)

Thus the defining characteristic of a primary group is its formation and maintenance by face-to-face communication.

# Secondary group subculture

A secondary group (e.g. a hospital) consists of a number of primary groups. The culture of each secondary group may be influenced not only by the configuration of subcultures that are active in its domain, but also by an overarching culture at the level of the whole institution. Thus the culture of an institution such as the NHS may be composed of a complex of interacting secondary cultures. This does not mean that secondary groups and institutions are merely the sums of their constituent primary and secondary groups:

> The standards of the primary groups do not develop in a vacuum; they develop within the general system of standards of the secondary groups in which they are incorporated.
> (Sprott, 1958, p. 21)

It is conventional to distinguish between 'natural' and 'artificial' primary groups, which differ from one another in at least two dimensions. The natural group, like a family, village or street, just grows by people coming to live there. This is quite different to the artificial formation of a focus group or a special committee. The work group falls between the two – it is relatively permanent in that it endures even if the membership changes, but it is formed for a specific purpose. It is arguably because of the need for regular rites of initiation, intensification and passage occasioned by a regularly changing membership, along with the functional importance of its communication with the secondary group, that the work group is such an interesting subject for study.

# Leadership

Leadership qualifies as a special type of subculture because its influence in the strategic affairs of organisations is considered to be so important. Furthermore, leadership impinges on all of the other subcultural elements of an organisation, as a demand for leadership can arise in any and all subcultures. As it is so important, we shall examine leadership in some detail.

Leadership studies have tended to be detached from other aspects of organisational research, with the notable exception of organisational culture, where it has received a good deal of attention from some scholars. Many authors have dealt with the personal traits and management styles of designated leaders. Others have tended to focus more on the contingencies and situations within which leaders (designated or not) tend to emerge. Healthcare organisations need effective leadership to guide them through the rocky shoals of economic scarcity, political expediency, and sea changes in patient demography, epidemiology, expectations and strategic policy. We shall briefly summarise the key phases of research into leadership, and relate them to organisational culture.

According to Stogdill:

> Leadership may be considered as the process (act) of influencing the activities of an organized group in its efforts toward goal setting and goal achievement.
>
> (Stogdill, 1950, p. 3)

The three elements that are contained in the above definition inform much of the research that followed Stogdill's influential work. Leadership is viewed as a process of inducing others to behave in certain desired ways, the process of influence is seen as occurring in a group setting, and the direction of influence is usually towards preconceived group goals (Bryman, 1996). Although this basic orientation towards leadership has remained fairly constant, analyses of the factors and resources available and deployed to exert influence in the process of leadership have varied considerably over the years. Stogdill refers to *leadership*, not to leaders. It was precisely that distinction between a quality, attribute, property or process of leadership and the notion of a natural-born leader that Selznick (1957) emphasised.

Up to the 1980s, research on leadership tended to focus on the logistical, communicational and social psychological problems that are faced by leaders in the process of goal achievement. However, during the 1980s a new definition of leadership evolved around the management of meaning (Smircich and Morgan, 1982) and symbolic action (Pfeffer, 1981). According to this view, leadership is about defining organisational realities, making sense of ambiguous situations and information, and persuading subordinates to adopt the leader's view of things:

> Leadership is seen as a process whereby the leader identifies for subordinates a sense of what is important – defining organizational reality for others. The leader gives a sense of direction and of purpose through the articulation of a compelling world-view.
>
> (Bryman, 1996, p. 276)

One source of confusion in leadership studies is the lack of a clear distinction between leadership and management, although Selznick (1957) attempted to make this distinction clear by linking a need for leadership to critical decision making. According to this view, leadership is not needed in the context of routine decisions, which can be made by administrators or managers. This distinction was developed by Zaleznik (1977) and Kotter (1990), who distinguished between management (which is concerned with the routine running of things) and leadership (which is concerned with such strategic concerns as an organisation's mission, identity and development). Thus the essential difference between leadership and management lies in the orientation to organisational change (Bryman, 1996). As change leaders need to engage the organisational culture – which can make or break most strategic initiatives – leadership came to be defined as 'symbolic leadership', and was closely tied to the strategic task of managing the organisational culture. These developments should be seen in the context of a long and continuing search for a Holy Grail of management. If one could only find some way of getting to employees' hearts and minds, it was thought, everything else in terms of effort, moral commitment and creativity would follow (Fox, 1985). As we shall now see, there has in fact been little consensus among scholars with regard to a proper definition of leadership or its role.

---

**Box 1.3**   The four stages of leadership theory and research (adapted from Bryman, 1996)

- The trait approach
- The style approach
- The contingency approach
- The new leadership approach

---

Bryman (1996) has divided the history of leadership theory and research into four main phases (*see* Box 1.3), each associated with a particular time period. The *trait approach* was dominant up to the 1940s, the *style approach* was prevalent from then until the 1960s, the *contingency approach* was favoured from the late 1960s to the early 1980s, and the *new leadership approach* has been prominent since the early 1980s. The influence–group–goal thematic cluster predominates in the first three of these phases. The following anatomy of leadership and its relationship to organisational culture is based on Bryman's cogent account.

# The trait approach

The trait approach is based on the belief that leaders are born, not made. It seeks to isolate essential leadership qualities in those who have achieved positions of power and influence. Many different traits have been investigated, including physical attributes (e.g. physique, height and appearance), innate abilities (e.g. intelligence and fluency of speech) and personality traits (e.g. conservatism, introversion–extroversion and self-confidence).

Reviews by Stogdill (1948, 1950, 1974), Gibb (1947) and Mann (1959) questioned the validity and consistency of trait research. Brown (1954) drew upon

Moreno's work on sociometry, and concluded that there are many varieties of leadership, which represent the diverse needs of community participants:

> It follows that there is no such thing as a 'natural' or 'universal' leader in the popular meaning of the phrase – a good leader is a man or woman who is most fitted to take charge in a given situation. Leadership is not a psychological trait which can be investigated as if it were a property of the individual – it is always a function of the situation and the nature of the group.
>
> (Brown, 1954, pp. 136–7)

# The style approach

Although trait research lingered on and even enjoyed something of a revival in a revised form in the late 1980s, from the late 1940s the focus shifted to leadership *behaviour*. Thus the emphasis switched from *selecting* natural leaders to fill future leadership positions to *preparing* and *training* individuals for leadership roles. Stogdill and others at Ohio State University conducted a large number of studies in the field. Their approach was to administer questionnaires to the subordinates of leaders, who in the early years tended to be in military organisations. Each subordinate was asked to indicate how well a statement about a leader's behaviour fitted the behaviour of his or her leader. The subordinates' scores were aggregated to give an overall score for each leader on each of a number of aspects of behaviour. Two main dimensions of leadership behaviour were emphasised, namely *consideration* and *initiating structure*. Consideration denotes a style of leadership that shows concern about subordinates as people, attracts trust and responsiveness from them and promotes camaraderie. Initiating structure denotes a style of leadership that defines in detail what subordinates are supposed to do. Leaders' scores on these two styles were then related to various outcome measures, such as group performance and subordinate job satisfaction. Early findings suggested that consideration was related to higher morale and job satisfaction among subordinates but lower levels of performance. Initiating structure was found to be associated with lower morale but better group performance. Later research tended to suggest that higher levels of both leadership styles were associated with better outcomes on all of the measures.

The Ohio studies were criticised on a number of grounds. Korman (1966) noted that their findings were plagued by inconsistent results. He also pointed out that insufficient attention was paid to the possibility that the effectiveness of leadership style might be contingent on the situation. The results of studies using experimental and longitudinal designs, by Lowin and Craig (1968) and Greene (1975) among others, tended to undermine the leadership–outcome inference. Furthermore, the almost exclusive focus on formally designated leaders came under attack for its neglect of informal leadership processes. The aggregation of subordinates' ratings ignored differences in the perceptions of leaders between subordinates. Finally, the validity of the Ohio scales was criticised in terms of the impact of subordinates' 'implicit leadership theories' on how they rated their leaders' behaviour. For example, Rush *et al.* (1977) showed that individuals' ratings of imaginary leaders were very similar to their ratings of real leaders, indicating that the Ohio research was probably measuring people's preconceptions of leadership, rather than their naive assessment of their actual leaders (Lord and Maher, 1991).

# The contingency approach

The contingency approach to leadership examines the situational variables that moderate the effectiveness of different types of leadership. It argues against notions of leadership as an essential quality that is held by certain individuals and not by others, or of leadership as a set of behaviours that can be learned and applied to any situation. Fiedler's contingency model of leadership (Fiedler, 1967, 1993; Fiedler and Garcia, 1987) is one of the best-known examples of this approach. At its core is the 'least preferred co-worker' (LPC) scale, which claims to measure the leadership orientation of individuals who complete it. Respondents are asked to describe the person whom they have least liked working with in terms of pairs of adjectives (e.g. pleasant–unpleasant, friendly–unfriendly, rejecting–accepting, distant–close). The results are scored, with higher scores indicating a positive view of the least preferred co-worker (pleasant, friendly, accepting, close, etc.) and lower scores indicating a negative view. Fiedler argues that people with high LPC scores are more relationship-motivated leaders, whereas people with low LPC scores are more task-motivated. From the results of numerous studies, Fiedler found that the effectiveness of relationship- and task-motivated leaders varied according to how favourable the situation was to the leader. This idea, which has since been termed *situational control*, has three components, namely leader–member relationships, task structure and position power. Fiedler found that task-orientated leaders were most effective in high-control and low-control situations, whereas relationship-orientated leaders performed best in moderate-control situations.

Fiedler's model has been criticised for its exclusive focus on situational control as the only situational factor, and there has been widespread disagreement about the model's validity. Like the Ohio studies, Fiedler's contingency approach examines formally designated leaders and virtually excludes informal leadership processes. Although contingency approaches still have their supporters, later research suggests that situational factors should not be allowed to eclipse entirely the characteristics of individuals fulfilling leadership roles. For example, Kennedy (1982) found that leaders with mid-range scores performed better than leaders with either low or high LPC scores, regardless of the levels of situational control. Podsakoff *et al.* (1984) found that the reward and punishment behaviour of leaders was associated with various measures of outcome, regardless of a range of situational factors examined.

# The new leadership approach

The 'new leadership' approaches which emerged in the 1980s coined a variety of terms to describe the type of leadership with which they were concerned. These included transformational leadership (Bass, 1985; Tichy and Devanna, 1986), charismatic leadership (House, 1977; Conger, 1989), visionary leadership (Sashkin, 1988; Westley and Mintzberg, 1989) and simply 'leadership' (Bennis and Nanus, 1985; Kotter, 1990). These labels share a common conception of leaders as managers of meaning, visionaries, and creators and interpreters of organisational symbols. The new leadership approach owes much to Burns's study of political leadership. Burns (1978) proposed a distinction between 'transactional leadership' (concerned with managing the exchange of effort and reward represented by the employment contract) and 'transforming leadership' – which later became 'transformational leadership' (concerned with an almost spiritual alliance between leaders and followers 'in a mutual and continuing pursuit of a higher purpose') (Burns, 1978, p. 20).

Burns's dichotomy was popularised by Peters and Waterman's bestseller *In Search of Excellence* (Peters and Waterman, 1982), which found that nearly all of the highly successful companies which they studied had been influenced by a transforming leadership at some stage in their development. In addition to its orientation towards the leader as a visionary manager of meaning, the new leadership approach has two other distinctive characteristics. First, its research is conducted on very senior leaders, such as chief executives of large multinational corporations, rather than on a range of middle managers, supervisors and others, as in the Ohio studies and Fiedler's research. Secondly, and unlike the trait, style or contingency approaches, qualitative case studies are utilised, including semi-structured interviews and documentary evidence.

With the exception of Bass and Alvolio (1990, 1993), the new leadership research suffers from similar weaknesses to previous approaches and also has some distinctive faults of its own. It concentrates on top leaders, has little to say about informal leadership processes, ignores the contextual factors which can constrain even the most visionary leaders (e.g. the type of business, technology, trading conditions, etc.) and is suspect in terms of validity. Peters and Waterman only visited high-performing organisations, so no comparison was made with leaders of less than excellent companies.

# Dispersed leadership

In addition to the focus by some new leadership research on heroic individual leaders at the highest organisational levels, several other streams of research into 'dispersed leadership' appeared during the 1990s. Manz and Sims (1991) and Sims and Lorenzi (1992) developed a new leadership paradigm dubbed 'super-leadership'. Super-leadership is about developing the leadership capacity in others in order to reduce their dependence on formal leaders and release their abilities and motivation. Katzenbach and Smith (1993) extolled the virtues of 'real teams', conceiving the leader to be a facilitator who cultivates the group and removes obstacles from its path.

# Leadership and organisational culture

Leadership has been a prominent theme in the work of some but by no means all writers on organisational culture. According to Schein, 'the unique and essential function of leadership is the manipulation of culture' (Schein, 1985, p. 317). Clarke (1970) and Pettigrew (1979) were interested in the lasting influence of the founder on new organisations and the continuities and sometimes dramatic changes that occurred over time. Trice and Beyer (1990) have distinguished between maintenance and innovative aspects of 'cultural leadership'. Innovation occurs when the founder creates a new culture or when a new leader attempts to replace an existing culture. Much of the new leadership research has tended to focus on situations where an imperative for organisational change is perceived. In these circumstances there is a perceived need to engage with the organisational culture, because it is regarded as the cohesive whole that binds the organisation together as a social system, because it is threatened by the change and can resist the organisation's transformation, and because radical change necessitates the formation of a new effective culture. This view is exemplified by Whipp's investigation of Jaguar and Hill Samuel in the UK, which concluded that a transformation of the organisation's culture was a prerequisite for radical strategic change. In their study of the links between organisational culture and performance, Kotter and Heskett (1992) saw leadership as necessary to change cultures in order to make them more adaptive to environmental change. According to this perspective, the key contribution of leadership to organisational culture is its 'value engineering' function. The leader is the one who defines the new reality, makes it meaningful, and persuades subordinates to 'buy into' the values that he or she envisages and prescribes.

Martin (1992) has defined three perspectives for examining leadership in relation to culture, namely the 'integration', 'differentiation' and 'fragmentation' perspectives. From the integration perspective, leadership is concerned with creating a consensus about the organisational culture such that everyone shares a similar vision, agrees on values and strives towards shared goals (Peters and Waterman, 1982; Schein, 1985, 1990; Trice and Beyer, 1990; Kotter and Heskett, 1992; Trice and Beyer, 1993). A variation on the integration perspective is provided by Alvesson (1992), who shows how managers in a Swedish computer consultancy firm have an integrative function by transmitting the organisation's culture, thus counteracting a tendency for the firm to splinter due to the decentralised and heterogeneous work of the consultants. In this case the leader's role is to transmit the culture, rather than to mould it. This case may be particularly relevant to dispersed health systems such as the NHS. In the NHS context of clinical governance, and the role of the National Institute for Clinical Excellence (NICE), there are similar requirements to transmit consistent narratives on quality, evidence-based practice and accountability to all sites around the UK.

From the differentiation perspective, culture is seen in terms of a lack of consensus across the organisation. This perspective draws particular attention 'to subcultural diversity and the resulting enclaves of consensus that form within the wider organisation' (Bryman, 1996, p. 285). Here the focus shifts from leadership that is exercised by individuals to leadership exercised by groups. This perspective addresses the otherwise neglected issue of informal leadership processes. Studies of informal organisation have examined the important role played by leaders of subcultures (Homans, 1950) and countercultures (Martin and Seihl, 1983), but this question has not been awarded the priority that it arguably deserves. The NHS and other health systems present examples of organisational cultures that are composed of a number of clearly definable subcultures (medical, managerial, nursing, therapeutic, etc.). Clearly, individuals do exercise leadership in subcultures, but subcultures may also exercise leadership over other subcultures, even to the extent of holding hegemonic influence over an organisational culture as a whole. In the NHS, a medical subculture has provided both subcultural and individual leadership, even after the introduction of general management. Clinical governance and numerous other policies that have been introduced in recent years embody a strategy to alter that status quo, partly by a revision of medical values (substitution of epidemiological evidence for case evidence) and the subordination of practice to a supra-medical administration. In the process of this change, a sharper focus is required on the analysis and implications of those shifts for the relative power of NHS subcultures. Failure to address this issue may lead to an entrenchment of the distinctive values and assumptions that support subcultures, with paralysing effects on organisational functioning and the achievement of change.

The differentiation perspective decentres leadership within an organisation's culture, but that does not imply any diminution of its role and importance. The main strengths of the differentiation perspective lie in signalling the possibility of a lack of consensus within an organisational culture, problematising the role of leadership as promoting such consensus, and highlighting a challenge to senior leaders about how to deal with, and perhaps actively manage, the balance of power between subcultures either via their leaders or by other means.

The fragmentation perspective views organisational culture as being suffused with ambiguity, confusion and uncertainty. This perspective offers little guidance to senior leaders who wish to implement cultural change, since it denies the possibility of influencing organisational culture to any significant extent (Martin, 1992; Bryman, 1996). There is of course a difference between an analysis of an organisational culture as fragmentary, and an assertion that all organisational cultures are *necessarily* fragmentary. We should not forget that the emergence of an organisational culture is closely related to the structural characteristics of an organisation by dint of its deliberate association of work groups — an observation that is of particular relevance to a subcultural analysis. Perhaps the most useful contribution made by the fragmentary approach is the finding that leaders can be sources of ambiguity in themselves (Tierney, 1989). Tierney (1987) shows how a new leader's actions can be consistently misunderstood and even seen to symbolise the opposite of the intended message. Any sign can be cynically interpreted, for example, as an attempt to exploit, seduce or beguile employees, and this effect alone demonstrates how difficult it can be to manage an organisational culture. It casts doubt on the basic assumption that culture is manageable. The fragmentation perspective views leaders' symbolic messages as equivocal, and considers that it is as important to observe their actual effects among the staff who receive them as it is to know the effect intended by the leader who transmits them.

# The consumption of culture

The fragmentary perspective is reinforced by a developing emphasis in research on how culture is *received*, by examining people's interpretations and creative 'use' or 'culture consumption' (Linstead and Grafton-Small, 1992). This approach can be seen in Hatch's critique (Hatch, 1993) of an ethnographic study of strategic change by the new president of a large US university (Gioia and Chittipeddi, 1991). Although he played an important role in initiating strategic change, the president's influence was contingent on how others represented and interpreted his efforts. Thus the outcome of his influence was unpredictable, because it depended on how others' interpretations affected cultural assumptions and expectations. The implication that Bryman draws from this approach to cultural leadership is that 'organizational members are not passive receptacles, but *imaginative consumers*, of leaders' visions and of manipulated cultural artefacts' (Bryman, 1996, p. 286).

We can extend the theme of cultural consumption to the public consumption of leaders' cultural influence. In the case of the NHS and other health systems, this implies an analysis of organisational culture as an arena in which forces of symbolic production and consumption combine to determine a culture that extends beyond the physical locations, boundaries and consciousness of the organisation as it is conventionally understood, and into the wider public domain. As Douglas and Isherwood (1979/1996) put it: 'Consumption is the very arena in which culture is fought over and licked into shape'. NHS culture is suffused throughout society, in the sense that its artefacts, espoused values and underlying assumptions are of concern to everyone. Few other institutions can be found whose spaces consumers penetrate as deeply or whose activities they participate so intimately in. There are relatively few private spaces in the NHS as compared with a factory or the Civil Service. The NHS is an intensely public organisation, and the public should be seen as active participants in its cultural life. Therefore we should begin to perceive and incorporate into the analysis a *public subculture* to the NHS whose influence on its formation, maintenance and change deserves to be more explicitly recognised and examined.

The role of leadership in organisational culture is an important area of theory and research. The narrative that we have offered, drawing on Bryman's (Bryman, 1996) and Martin's (Martin, 1992) analyses, is one in which an initially simplistic view of leaders as culture builders is followed by more subtle perspectives of leadership as a distributed and even fragmentary phenomenon. There are two caveats to be added to this account. The first is that most of what we have discussed was articulated, albeit in different terms, by earlier scholars such as Brown (1954) and Selznick (1957). Therefore there is another sense in which scholarship in this area has made only modest advances. Secondly, there are clear avenues down which much more substantial progress could be made. A view of leadership as being distributed among groups, rather than being simplistically located only at the apexes of organisational and divisional structures, recognises that leadership is a complex, dynamic and ambiguous phenomenon. This analysis can be extended to a hypothesis that the traits and behaviour of leaders may not be located in individuals, groups or even subcultures *per se*, but rather they denote a range of effects that, like subcultures, traverse throughout organisations, health systems such as the NHS, and even society at large.

This trajectory leads us on to the even more uncertain ground of post-modernist, deconstructivist and post-structuralist thinking. Here we can only deal with these ideas briefly and speculatively, which is to belie their growing importance and potential for leadership studies and organisational cultural analysis in general. A postmodern perspective on leadership might deny that any overall patterns of leadership behaviour exist beyond *narratives* of leadership. According to this view, a unitary or 'grand narrative' of leadership belongs to an outdated, modernist conception of industrial development as expressing general laws of capital, labour and technological and administrative science (Burrell, 1996). This progressive global perspective has been disrupted by a postmodern perspective of multiple local narratives of leadership (Lyotard, 1984).

A deconstructionist perspective on leadership (after Jacques Derrida) might conceive of organisational culture as a kind of writing, a text that is co-written by all participants. According to this view, the leader is not the sole 'author' of a leadership role. Equally important are all of the readers (subordinates and others) who 'read' that leadership role and behaviour and find them meaningful in different ways. From such a perspective, no one assessment of a leader, including his or her own self-assessment, is privileged over that of anyone else. However, each has one thing in common with all of the other authors/readers, which is that such meaning as they find in a leader's role is determined by favouring certain interpretations over others, which are repressed. The 'text' of leadership contains many possible meanings and interpretations, of which some are selected and others are opposites forced into the background. This leads to an interesting effect. A repressed meaning continually reasserts itself, such that leadership is a contested terrain that is fought over at every level of construction and interpretation.

A post-structuralist perspective on leadership is perhaps the hardest to understand because it emerges from a completely different way of thinking about things. At its heart is a radical disbelief in the centrality or permanence of the human condition. According to this view, leadership is not an essentially human trait or activity, but rather it is an expression of certain supra-human forces, of which human nature and organisation are also expressions. According to this view, there is nothing that is essentially human. The human condition and organisation are expressions of the forces of production driven by the energy of desire (Deleuze and Guattari, 1983). There are no limits to leadership attributes or styles. According to this perspective, a true leader is one who creates roles, values, interpretations and directions. There can be no model leadership role here, as anyone who needs a model is not a leader.

These examples of postmodern, deconstructionist and post-structuralist perspectives on leadership might appear tangential to the role of 'real' leaders in 'real' organisations. We mention them here because they indicate themes in contemporary economic, social and organisational research, which will over the coming years become perspectives of great importance and reality. Moreover, it is important to understand that these perspectives do not emerge from the mere fancy of philosophers, but from investigations into problematic assumptions about what is real, the role of knowledge, the practical conduct of economic, social and organisational life, and the nature of culture.

# How organisational cultures change

The diversity of models for understanding organisational culture change reflects a lack of theoretical consensus surrounding definitions of organisational culture and processes of organisational change (Brown, 1995). We have explored a dichotomy between researchers who have approached organisational culture as an organisational *variable* and those who define organisation *as* culture. These basic approaches have different implications for organisational change, both accidental and managed. Conceived as a variable, organisational culture appears to be capable of natural variation and purposive manipulation, whereas organisational culture as the expression or production of social organisation suggests a strong sense of autonomy and unpredictability. In addition to the five models suggested by Smircich (1983), theorists tend to define the 'essence' of culture differently. For example, Kilmann (1984) defines organisational culture in terms of norms, whereas Lundberg (1985) and Schein (1985, 1990) define the 'essence' of culture as the deeply held assumptions that shape norms, values and behaviour. Deeply held assumptions of which the holder is largely unaware present a greater analytical challenge and greater resistance to change than norms, which can be more easily identified and challenged. Whatever their views on the 'essence' of culture, most current theorists agree that organisational cultures tend to be highly resistant to change.

Brown (1995) has identified five models of culture change (*see* Box 1.4). All of these models define culture in terms of deeply held beliefs, values or assumptions.

---

**Box 1.4**   Five models of organisational culture change (adapted from Brown, 1995)

- *Lundberg's model*, based on earlier learning-cycle models of organisational change, emphasises external environmental factors as well as internal characteristics of organisations.
- *Dyer's model* posits that the perception of crisis in conjunction with a leadership change is required for culture change to occur.
- *Schein's model*, based on a simple life-cycle framework, posits that different culture change mechanisms are associated with different stages in an organisation's development.
- *Gagliardi's model* suggests that only incremental culture change can properly be described as a form of organisational change.
- *A composite model*, based on the ideas of Lewin, Beyer and Trice and Isabella, provides some insights into the microprocesses of culture change.

---

# Lundberg's model

Lundberg argues that in order for change to occur, certain external and internal factors must be present. The two external enabling conditions are *domain forgiveness*, which refers to the degree of threat to an organisation (e.g. competition, scarcity or abundance of resources, environmental stability or instability). The more forgiving the environment, the more likely it is that change will occur, because the risk of change will be lower than in a less forgiving environment. The second external condition is *organisational-domain* congruence. If the degree of congruence between the organisation and the domain is too low or too high, then change might be either too threatening or unnecessary. Change is more likely to occur when there is a moderate degree of congruence.

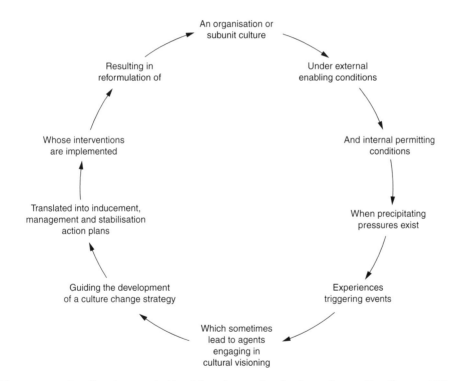

**Figure 1.2** Lundberg's organisational learning cycle of culture change (Lundberg, 1985).

Lundberg also identifies the following four *internal permitting conditions* that allow change:

1 sufficient change resources (e.g. money, managerial time and energy)
2 system readiness (i.e. a collective sense that people are willing to change)

3 co-ordinative and integrative mechanisms that facilitate communication and control
4 a stable leadership team with sufficient awareness, vision, power and communication skills to guide culture change.

In addition, Lundberg postulates the following four types of *precipitating pressures* that will make organisational members more likely to change:

1 atypical performance demands (e.g. to be more productive)
2 stakeholder pressures (which might come from the public, the Government, unions, etc.)
3 pressures resulting from organisational growth or contraction
4 a perception of crisis (e.g. financial losses or large debts).

Lundberg postulates one further condition that must be present before cultural change can be initiated, namely a *triggering event*. The following five classes of triggering event are posited:

1 environmental disasters (e.g. recession)
2 environmental opportunities (e.g. technological breakthroughs)
3 internal revolutions (e.g. a change in senior management)
4 external revolutions (e.g. nationalisation)
5 managerial crisis (e.g. a serious blunder by senior executives).

If the trigger event catches organisational leaders by surprise, they may respond by initiating a process of enquiry. This will involve clarifying the existing culture and envisioning alternatives. Lundberg terms this *cultural visioning*.

Success in establishing a new culture depends on the new vision being transformed into a *culture change strategy* that is implemented through action plans. The change strategy should determine three important factors:

1 the *pace of change* (will change be quick or slow?)
2 the *scope of change* (how radical will the change be?)
3 the *time span* (over what period will change occur?).

Three specific forms of action planning are required:

1 *inducement action plans* that heighten system readiness for change and counter resistance to change
2 *management action plans* that enable members to redefine the culture in line with the culture change strategy
3 *stabilisation action plans* that reinforce the changes and ensure their persistence over time.

These plans might include discrediting dominant myths and legends, rewriting the organisation's history and introducing new metaphors. They may also involve the use of external consultants, refashioning the organisation's identity, redesigning training programmes and revising recruitment and selection criteria.

This multi-variable model represents some of the complexity of organisational change. Lundberg emphasises two further points. First, he highlights the importance of engaging all levels of culture, from artefacts to underlying assumptions through the change strategy. Secondly, he points out that continuous, repeated, multiple interventions are more likely to succeed than single short-term interventions. However, Lundberg is sceptical about the possibility of managing organisational culture change:

> The complexity of the phenomena of organizational culture, the inherent difficulty of impacting deep levels of cultural meaning, and the vision required for designing and sequencing the multiple interventions needed suggest that managing culture is not often likely, even if it is possible. ... Yet organizational culture change does happen.
>
> (Lundberg, 1985, p. 183)

## Evaluation

Lundberg's model acknowledges the complexity of organisational change, including its contingency on external and internal conditions. It also recognises the multiple layers of culture that exist and need to be tackled by a change strategy, and the presence of multiple subcultures. All of this makes it extremely difficult to effect planned culture change. However, the model is rather mechanistic, failing to acknowledge fully the dynamism and uncertainty of the relationship between cause and effect in organisational life. It also fails to address the political forces (e.g. 'board wars') at play in the organisation, and the influence of key individuals and groups on culture change. The causality between conditions such as domain forgiveness and change is open to question. Taking business process re-engineering (BPR) as an example, most reports of BPR in US healthcare settings state that change occurred in response to completely unforgiving environmental imperatives, namely the spread of managed care. This contradicts Lundberg's notion that organisational culture will not change in the face of environmental risk. The relationship between domain forgiveness and organisational domain congruence is also unclear. Thus it is an interesting but limited view of only some of the organisational processes that precede and promote culture change.

## Dyer's cycle of cultural evolution

Dyer's framework (Dyer, 1985) is derived from the case histories of five large US companies (General Motors, Levi Strauss, National Cash Register, the Balfour

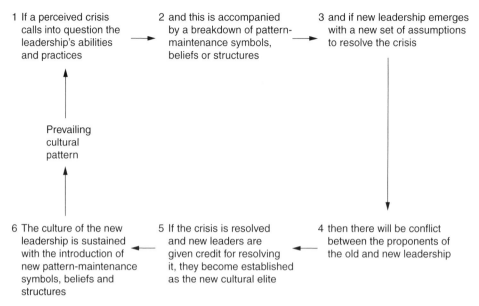

1 If a perceived crisis calls into question the leadership's abilities and practices

2 and this is accompanied by a breakdown of pattern-maintenance symbols, beliefs or structures

3 and if new leadership emerges with a new set of assumptions to resolve the crisis

Prevailing cultural pattern

6 The culture of the new leadership is sustained with the introduction of new pattern-maintenance symbols, beliefs and structures

5 If the crisis is resolved and new leaders are given credit for resolving it, they become established as the new cultural elite

4 then there will be conflict between the proponents of the old and new leadership

**Figure 1.3**   The cycle of cultural evolution in organisations (Dyer, 1985).

Company and the Brown Corporation*). It is based on a definition of culture consisting of four levels, namely artefacts, perspectives (rules and norms), values and assumptions. Although it is presented as a linear cycle (*see* Figure 1.3), Dyer acknowledges that the stages can overlap or occur simultaneously.

1 In the first stage of the cycle, the leadership's abilities and current practices are called into question. Usually this is triggered by an adverse event, which creates a perception of crisis that members believe cannot be solved using current methods. Dyer suggests that environmental change (e.g. recession) is the usual cause. Healthcare examples of crises could include the challenge posed to conventional health insurance by the emergence of managed care in the USA, and the crisis in public confidence caused by the recent series of NHS scandals in the UK.

2 The perception of crisis causes a breakdown in what Dyer terms the pattern-maintenance symbols, beliefs and structures – the means by which a culture is sustained. That breakdown is necessary in order to make way for a new culture. The symbols, beliefs and structures can include dominant leaders, reward systems and all system-supportive beliefs. In the NHS culture such a breakdown in pattern-maintenance symbols, beliefs and structures can be seen in the gradual erosion of the power of physicians by developments in health policy, management, epidemiology and patients' rights.

---

* The Brown Corporation is a pseudonym (Brown, 1995, p. 125).

3 However, a breakdown in the culture's supportive symbols, beliefs and structures is not a sufficient condition for culture change. The promulgation of an alternative set of artefacts, approaches, values and assumptions is also required.
4 The arrival of the new leadership sparks conflict between supporters of the old and new cultures. Those who are unable to accept the new order may have to leave the organisation or be transferred to powerless positions. This might provoke a counter-attack by the old order, which the new order should anticipate and swiftly quash, otherwise conflict could drag on for years.
5 In the conflict resolution stage, the new leadership elite must deal with resentment and resistance caused by their new practices. The new leader must be credited with successfully solving these crises, which increases that individual's powers and reduces the power of reactionary rivals.

In order to embed the new culture in the organisation, the new leadership must then begin to create new pattern-maintenance symbols, beliefs and structures. In addition to recruiting people who are supportive of the new order and weeding out non-conformists, the past history of the organisation is typically reinterpreted. The old leadership is seen to have failed because it was weak and unprofessional, all of which serves as justification for the new regime.

According to Dyer's model, then, organisational cultural change comes out of a crisis that affects the old leadership, as well as the effectiveness of a new leadership in taking cultural control:

> According to the model described here, the most important decision in culture change concerns the selection of a new leader inasmuch as a new leader who enters an organization during a period of crisis has unique opportunities to transform the organization's culture by bringing and embedding new artefacts, perspectives, values, and assumptions into the organization. Leaders do indeed appear to be the creators and transmitters of culture.
>
> (Dyer, 1985, p. 223)


## Evaluation

An advantage of Dyer's model over many other theoretical models is that its two essential conditions for cultural transformation, namely crisis and new leadership, are relatively easy to identify and test in organisational settings. It also usefully emphasises the importance of leadership in organisational culture and change. However, the framework can be criticised for its overly simplistic view of culture change processes. The roles of the majority of participants in an organisational culture are eclipsed in favour of a monothematic focus on innovative leadership. Yet the importance of culture to organisational change surely arises from the recognition that culture is sufficiently powerful to defeat the transformational efforts of any leaders, old or new. As Sir Peter Parker ruefully remarked while he was Chairman of British Rail, changing organisational culture is like trying to run through a field of treacle. In an earlier section on leadership we examined several different definitions and considered alternatives to the trait approach. These included informal leadership, situational leadership and leadership by groups. These alternative conceptions of leadership appear to be applicable to large healthcare organisations consisting of complexes of subcultures. If so, we would expect alternative artefacts, values, approaches and assumptions to be promulgated by subcultures, as well as by individual leaders. Examples of changes in subcultural leadership might include the reintroduction of matrons, signalling to other groups that senior nurses are a force to be reckoned with. Other examples might include clinical governance, which allocates new accountabilities for the quality of care delivered, with implications for the autonomy of practitioners, and the National Institute for Clinical Excellence (NICE), which functions to rationalise the availability of treatments on evidential rather than commercial grounds. These and other developments explicitly promote an epidemiological culture to replace a gradually discredited culture that has been based on traditional non-scientific methods of healthcare. However, they are arguably the result of generalised and diffuse movements in healthcare and research, not just of the efforts of individual leaders.

It is odd that Dyer should term his model 'evolutionary', when it is quite clearly *revolutionary*, positing as it does the overthrow of an old, failing regime by a new, stronger one. Dyer's analysis of culture change appears to be similar to Kuhn's theory of scientific revolutions (Kuhn, 1970), except that according to Kuhn the supporters of the old paradigm will labour on until they retire. Owing to their strong subcultural influence, and the projected shortage of doctors, a slow, Kuhnian revolution in NHS culture appears to be more plausible than Dyer's sudden coup scenario. By contrast, the rise of capitation in the USA does appear to constitute a revolution. However, it remains to be seen whether capitation will permanently displace the old order of fee for service.

One suspects that, like most accounts of victorious revolution, Dyer's model is useful for rewriting organisational history in the words of the victors, but less applicable to a detailed analysis of organisational cultural change. The NHS frequently has crises which strong leadership would doubtless help to resolve. However, the notion that a wholesale transformation of the organisation's culture could be achieved by replacing one leadership with another is not credible. We have only to look at the history of Britain's railways since their privatisation to see that a revolutionary change of leadership and ownership is probably not the best way forward, and can be even more disastrous than the original 'crisis'. New leadership is not the answer if the old leadership was not at fault. Dyer's model fails to ask a crucial and rather obvious question about the *causes* of crises in organisations. In answering that question, it may be found that culture is a factor, but possibly only in the sense of its mediation of other more easily manipulable variables, such as finance and financial control, remuneration and career structures, political interference, recruitment and retention, the focus of care, occupational identity and interaction, and so on.

# Schein's life-cycle model

Schein's life-cycle model of organisational culture change (Schein, 1985) suggests that organisations undergo distinct stages of development, each of which is associated with a different culture serving different functions and susceptible to change in different ways. These stages are *birth and early growth, organisational midlife* and *organisational maturity* (*see* Table 1.1).

## Birth and early growth

During this stage the cultural emphasis is on socialisation and cohesion. Mechanisms of change include natural evolution, the involvement of outside consultants in 'clinical' therapy to guide change, recruiting specific individuals to engineer change (evolution through hybrids), and revolutionary change by recruiting new leaders to steer the young organisation through crises.

Managed revolution involves conflict with the older culture, and scepticism, resistance and sabotage are all likely. Eventually a dominant view forms about whether the new regime has been successful or not. In the latter case the outsiders are likely to be forced out.

## Organisational midlife

In this phase the organisation is well established and the developmental instabilities are replaced by strategic choices with regard to growth, diversification and acquisitions. The culture of the organisation is fully formed and embedded in its routines and structures. Strong subcultures may have developed, making a deep understanding of the organisational culture both difficult and necessary for change. Mechanisms of change in organisational midlife include planned change and organisational development, technological seduction, scandal and explosion of myths, and incrementalism.

**Table 1.1:**   The different stages of Schein's life-cycle model of organisational culture

| Growth stage | Function of culture | Mechanism of change |
| --- | --- | --- |
| Birth and early growth<br>• Founder domination, possibly family domination | • Culture is a distinctive competence and source of identity<br>• Culture is the 'glue' that holds the organisation together<br>• Organisation strives towards greater integration and clarity<br>• Heavy emphasis on socialisation as evidence of commitment | 1 Natural evolution<br>2 Self-guided evolution through therapy<br>3 Managed evolution through hybrids<br>4 Managed 'revolution' through outsiders |
| *Succession phase* | • Culture becomes battleground between conservatives and liberals<br>• Potential successors are judged on whether they will preserve or change cultural elements | |
| Organisational midlife<br>• New product development<br>• Vertical integration<br>• Geographical expansion<br>• Acquisitions, mergers | • Cultural integration declines as new subcultures are spawned<br>• Crisis of identity, loss of key goals, values and assumptions<br>• Opportunity to manage direction of cultural change | 5 Planned change and organisational development<br>6 Technological seduction<br>7 Change due to scandal and explosion of myths<br>8 Incrementalism |
| Organisational maturity<br>• Maturity of markets<br>• Internal stability or stagnation<br>• Lack of motivation to change | • Culture becomes a constraint on innovation<br>• Culture preserves the glories of the past, so is valued as a source of self-esteem, defence | 9 Coercive persuasion<br>10 Turnaround<br>11 Reorganisation, destruction and rebirth |
| *Transformation option* | • Culture change is necessary and inevitable, but not all elements of culture can or must change<br>• Essential elements of culture must be identified and preserved<br>• Culture change can be managed or simply allowed to evolve | |

*(continued)*

**Table 1.1:**   (*continued*)

| Growth stage | Function of culture | Mechanism of change |
|---|---|---|
| *Destruction option*<br>• Bankruptcy and reorganisation<br>• Takeover and reorganisation<br>• Merger and assimilation | • Culture changes at basic levels<br>• Culture changes through massive replacement of key individuals | |

*Planned change and organisational development*

Schein (1985, 1999) defines organisational culture on three levels, namely artefacts, values and assumptions. Artefacts are the material signs that we can see, hear or otherwise sense when we enter the organisation (its distinctive architecture, behaviour, symbols, etc.). Values are the espoused rationale for how the organisation does what it does (e.g. the primacy of care and consideration for patients in the NHS). Assumptions are those values that have become so embedded in the culture that they are taken for granted. According to Schein, the basic methodology for assisting with organisational culture change involves looking for discrepancies between observed artefacts and espoused values. These, he observes, are usually explicable in terms of underlying assumptions that provide the basic substrate on which observable aspects of the culture are built. For example, one might perceive a discrepancy in NHS culture between patient-centred care (espoused value) and the long waiting-lists for some consultations and operations (artefacts). This could (hypothetically) be explained in terms of deeply held assumptions about professional status and personal income, about fraternity and solidarity within occupational groups, and about contempt for patients who appear to be unwilling to preserve their own health. Digging deeper still, an assumption might be found that patients are actually a kind of currency of exchange between practitioners, sustaining the professional interests of the latter but not necessarily meriting their consideration as social equals.

A recent formal visit to a New York healthcare facility provides what at first glance might seem a trivial example. During the visit, one of the authors of this book listened to senior staff espouse a philosophy of high levels of commitment and dedication to their patient population, and a belief in the value of organisational culture renewal. However, during the ensuing tour it was observed that the television in the waiting-room was faulty, or at least not properly tuned in, making it impossible for waiting patients to watch it, although some of them were trying to do so to pass the time. We do not know the significance of that discrepancy, and it is pointless to speculate in abstract, but unless the fault was very recent, it may have held some potential for discovering something significant about the organisation's culture. According to Schein, we should try to uncover the underlying assumptions that explain discrepancies between sincerely held beliefs and any artefacts that appear to contradict them. The badly tuned television set and the consequent frustration felt by some patients might have triggered an inquiry into institutional values relating to the social processes of care, in possible contrast to the value of equitable access articulated by the senior staff.

Planned change and organisational development involve facilitating culture change by analysing and bringing to the surface the values and assumptions of the dominant culture and subcultures. This process is seen as a way of 'unfreezing' the culture by providing mutual insight and developing commitment to superordinate organisational goals. It assumes that conflict between the dominant culture and subcultures within the organisation is a decisive spur to change.

*Technological seduction*
The introduction of new technology can be another stimulus to culture change by causing new patterns of social interaction, changing the nature of tasks and roles (consider the changes in medical imaging technology that have occurred over the last 20 years), and threatening the power bases of individuals who are affected by new technologies. Computerisation of medical information, from diagnostic techniques to pathology, has been a major change in recent decades, and promises to be matched by new developments in genetics. Many large organisations have had great difficulty in assimilating computerisation in a coherent and cost-effective way, and the NHS is an outstanding example of this failure. The organisational culture is one obstacle to this assimilation. People who are used to conceiving of a task in one habitual way can find it very difficult to conceive of that task being performed using entirely different techniques and knowledge bases. In addition, the fast pace of change and inherent redundancy of computer technologies pose difficulties to purchasers and system designers. It remains to be seen how well the NHS and other healthcare systems will cope with a genetic revolution.

*Change due to scandal and explosion of myths*
These are extreme cases of the artefact–value discrepancies mentioned earlier. The Bristol paediatric heart surgery tragedy is the most outstanding of these scandals to have occurred in the NHS in recent years (Kennedy, 2001). It is to be hoped that discrepancies between artefacts (dead and injured children, surgical group-think, 'whistle-blowing' taboo) and values (high moral commitment to the care of sick children) of this severity will lead to the examination of underlying assumptions and cultural change in the NHS.

*Incrementalism*
This refers to Quinn's description (Quinn, 1978) of how leaders actually hope to implement strategies. Incrementalism is a gradual process whereby one's

daily decisions will, if informed by a long-term desire for change, steer the organisation in that direction in the long term. In the NHS this is probably a view that is commonly held by clinicians – that by improving their knowledge and skills over the course of their careers, they will realise an inexorable progress towards better patient care. The new order of evidence-based medicine stands as a critique of medical incrementalism by trying to bring about a global revolution in the forms of scientific knowledge and information that guide healthcare practice.

## Organisational maturity

Other aspects of NHS culture fit into the maturity phase, in which the distinctive change mechanisms are coercive persuasion, turnaround, and reorganisation, destruction and rebirth.

### Coercive persuasion

Although it appears to be a harsh approach, there are some arguments in favour of forcing through cultural change, particularly in situations where employees have no alternative but to accept the new regime due to a tight labour market. Some cultures may be so intransigent that more subtle change processes have little chance of succeeding. The direct approach is also less covert and manipulative than the type of ideological warfare summoned by Dyer, which could be advantageous in the face of a sceptical, suspicious or cynical workforce. Sometimes a crisis calls for decisive action, and delay could threaten the organisation's very existence. In such cases the first duty of leaders is to keep the organisation afloat by whatever legal means are available. It could also be argued that if an organisational culture does emerge spontaneously from the sociotechnical milieu, as some researchers believe, then leaders should focus mainly on changing the technical organisation, and let the culture take care of itself. It should be added that forcing change is more likely to be successful if it is led by individuals who are highly skilled at persuasion.

### Turnaround

As the name suggests, this category involves transforming the failing organisation into a success story. John Harvey Jones' television series, *Troubleshooter*, exemplifies this approach. It requires an excellent grasp of all of the main aspects of business, and Schein claims that it is the leader's ability to coerce that will make or break a successful turnaround. To be successful in large organisations, culture change by turnaround implies that one person can effectively manipulate the controls of the organisation by implementing clear lines of responsibility and accountability. It is difficult to see how, in an extremely large and complex organisation such as the NHS, this level of control would be possible. It would be interesting to compare the extent of centralised control in the NHS with that in other large health systems, such as the Veterans' Administration or Kaiser Permanente.

*Reorganisation, destruction and rebirth*
Although Schein has little to say about this mechanism, it has become popular in the form of business process re-engineering (BPR). Mainly in response to managed care, many US hospitals and health systems have re-engineered themselves in a drastic attempt to adapt to the new healthcare market environment. BPR in its extreme form is a high-risk strategy – the organisational equivalent of a bone-marrow transplant. Because it involves destruction of the old organisational structure and culture prior to the introduction of the new arrangements, failure of BPR can spell death to the organisation. Fortunately, many so-called BPR programmes are less ambitious than the label implies. It has been estimated that by the early 1990s, 60% of US companies had attempted BPR, and that 70% of these had failed. BPR is closely linked to computerisation, obvious candidates being insurance companies converting to direct telesales. The most publicised BPR project in the NHS has been conducted at the Leicester Royal Infirmary Trust (McNulty and Ferlie, 2002). However, the term 'BPR' was later dropped from that programme, which has been criticised for selective reporting of results. Such high-risk change strategies are not generally appropriate for the NHS, which does not operate in a competitive market.

# Evaluation

Schein's perspective on organisational culture change recognises the difficulties involved to a greater extent than most other authors. As a psychologist and organisational consultant, Schein has adopted a 'clinical' rather than descriptive approach, drawing upon a strong anthropomorphic analogy of the organisation as a patient. Although there is some analytical and diagnostic value in the developmental stages that underpin Schein's model, it is unclear whether real organisations fit comfortably within them. The NHS as a whole appears to have the characteristics of both midlife and maturity, while new organisational forms such as primary care trusts will display some of the characteristics of birth and early growth. Schein's attitude towards organisational culture may be summarised as a recommendation that we work *with* it rather than *against* it. Faced with an organisation like the NHS, this is surely sound advice. However, in order to work with NHS culture, we first have to understand it.

# Gagliardi's model

Gagliardi's conception of organisational culture (Gagliardi, 1986) is similar to those of Lundberg, Dyer and Schein. He sees the essence of culture as the unconscious assumptions that are expressed in conscious values and material artefacts. However, his framework for culture change differs in that it advocates the view that this change occurs incrementally, not radically. Gagliardi argues that there are four phases in the development of an organisational value.

1  A leader defines objectives and evaluates tasks in accordance with specific beliefs. Although these beliefs might not be shared, the leader has the power to orient those under his control in the direction that he or she desires.
2  The belief is confirmed by experience and comes to be shared by all members of the organisation.
3  Employees turn their attention away from the effects of belief, coming instead to focus dogmatically on the belief as the cause of desirable effects.
4  Finally, the value comes to be shared unquestioningly and unconsciously by all concerned. Gagliardi terms this *idealisation,* in which a belief is *emotionally transfigured* (i.e. held on emotional rather than rational grounds). In Schein's terms, the value has become an assumption.

Gagliardi states that the need for large-scale change in an organisation is rarely perceived by those who are deeply involved in its culture, and is more likely to be seen by members of countercultures or by outsiders. Culture change therefore requires a change of leadership, from outside the dominant culture. Gagliardi distinguishes between cultural revolution, in which the old firm dies in order to be replaced by a new firm, and an incremental model of culture change (*see* Figure 1.4).

According to Gagliardi's model, an organisation's failure to cope with certain problems does not mean that the old culture needs to be destroyed, but rather that it has to expand its range of responses by incorporating new values. If the organisation then experiences success, the idealisation process will lead to the new values being subscribed to on emotional grounds and becoming assumptions in their turn. Tensions are resolved by appeals to reconciliation myths promulgated by the leadership. These myths convince people that the organisation's success is due to new practices, even though it might really be due to causes unconnected with the new ways of doing things:

> In cultural change, then, the role of the leader is, above all, to create conditions under which success can visibly be achieved, even if only in a limited or partial way, and to rationalize positive events after they have happened, even if accidental ... . A leader does not reinterpret past history to justify retrospectively his own proposals, nor does he go against existing myths; rather, he reinterprets the recent past and present in such a way that he promotes the insertion of new emergent values into the hierarchy of current

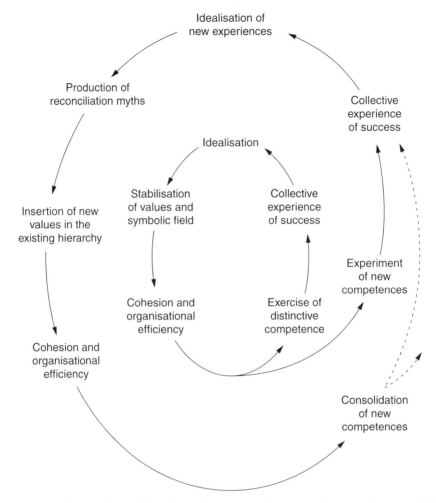

**Figure 1.4** Gagliardi's model: cultural change as an incremental process (Brown, 1995, p. 104).

operational ones, and encourages the birth of new myths which are superimposed on the old ones and reconcile new contradictions.

(Gagliardi, 1986, p. 132)

## *Evaluation*

Gagliardi's model of cultural change is interesting for two main reasons. First, it affirms the possibility of gradual change without the wholesale upset and cost of a revolutionary break in culture. Secondly, it provides insights into the pragmatic and often intuitive methods by which successful leaders may convert the inherent ambiguity of meaning of organisational events into clear (although possibly specious) attributions of cause and effect. They do this by shaping events into arguments in order to promote values and expand the competences of the organisation. On the negative side, Gagliardi's model sets great store on the irrational dimension of organisational life, but fails to address the obstacles that are presented to value engineering by scepticism and cynicism at all levels of an organisation.

# Understanding culture change: Lewin, Beyer and Trice, and Isabella

The final model of organisational change discussed by Brown (1995) is a compilation model based on the ideas of Lewin (1952) as modified by Schein (1964), Beyer and Trice (1988) and Isabella (1990). The framework examines the cultural processes associated with organisational culture change and adaptation in more detail than do the previous models. The framework (*see* Table 1.2) adopts Lewin's division of change into three phases, namely unfreezing, change and refreezing. Each phase is associated with certain rites, some of which we have already encountered in Brown's description of occupational cultures (Brown, 1954), and with a particular cognitive state.

## *Unfreezing*

Unfreezing begins when some leaders perceive a need for change, typically in response to negative events such as declining profitability. This information induces guilt anxiety, encouraging individuals to be more receptive to ideas

**Table 1.2:**  Understanding organisation culture change: three related domains (Brown, 1995)

| Contextual domain | Social domain | Cognitive domain |
|---|---|---|
| Unfreezing mechanisms | Rites of questioning and destruction<br>Rites of rationalisation and legitimation | Anticipation |
| Change | Rites of degradation and conflict<br>Rites of passage and enhancement | Confirmation<br>Culmination |
| Refreezing mechanisms | Rites of integration and conflict reduction | Aftermath |

about change. However, the felt need to change might be a localised phenomenon, unless it is cascaded down and across the organisation.

The unfreezing rites are *rites of questioning and destruction* and *rites of rationalisation and legitimation*. Rites of questioning and destruction formally challenge the established order of an organisation by presenting evidence that individuals or systems are failing to perform adequately. These rites take the form of presentations designed both to inform and to persuade, usually as part of an 'advertising campaign'. Other rites of questioning and destruction include bringing in external consultants, whose arm's-length perspective allows them to identify and criticise failing systems and practices. Consultants can act as catalysts for change by stimulating debate and questioning basic organisational assumptions. Rites of rationalisation and legitimation sensitise people to the significance of proposed changes by providing explanations as to why they are needed. Sensitising explanations legitimate the new thinking, making it appear necessary and acceptable. They also promote commitment to the proposed change programme. Rites of rationalisation and legitimation usually begin at senior management level, after which internal advocates of change are trained as trainers and this pattern is repeated down and across the organisation.

At the same time, employees typically suffer intense psychological stress induced by their *anticipation* (Isabella, 1990). During this phase people discuss the proposed changes, exchange rumours and hearsay, and generally build up pictures of what is going to happen, based on incomplete information. Unnecessary delay in giving information to employees about a change programme and the probable effects on their personal circumstances is common, and serves to increase their suffering.

# Change

During this phase, where the actual culture change occurs, there are two further associated rites, namely *rites of degradation and conflict* and *rites of passage and enhancement*. Rites of degradation and conflict constitute attacks on the old order. Rites of degradation include replacing staff who do not acknowledge the need for change with new staff who support the new order. Constructive conflict situations may be deliberately set up. For example, a powerful task force may be appointed to overcome resistance and sweep changes through, challenging the authority of reactionaries. Other rites of degradation and conflict include the introduction of new targets, milestones and performance indicators. These serve to legitimate the new order by instilling new objectives and values, thereby eroding the objectives, values and relevance of the old order. Rites of passage and enhancement are designed to instil a sense of identification with and belonging to the new order. This helps to reduce resistance to change (by providing a social incentive to join the in-group), broaden the base of support for the new order and encourage ownership of the process of change. Education and training play a prominent role, together with the promotions and job titles that reflect the new order. During this phase, individuals progress through two further cognitive states, which Isabella (1990) has termed confirmation and culmination. Once individuals have received adequate information, they will try to make sense of events using traditional explanations and previous experiences. This tendency to understand the new order by using old heuristics is termed the confirmation period. It helps to explain why some individuals and groups are unable to understand fully the changes that are being sought by the programme, by locating conflicting assumptions or paradigms upon which the changes are interpreted. Only when the deficiencies of the old assumptions have been clarified can participants progress to the culmination stage, in which the changes required are fully understood in their proper context.

## Refreezing

During the refreezing phase, individuals seek to reduce the uncertainty and instability in their work tasks and relationships that have been engendered by the change programme, and they settle into a more predictable modus operandi. This involves redefining the role and functions required of them and learning to work efficiently with new systems and groups of colleagues. During this phase the new cultural values become embedded as underlying assumptions.

Refreezing also has its associated rites, namely *rites of integration and conflict reduction*. These bring coherence to the organisation and reduce conflicts and rivalry between groups and departments. Rites of integration and conflict reduction consolidate the new order and raise morale. Praise from senior leaders, refresher training courses, group rituals and other rites contribute to this phase. They also encourage a cognitive shift to a state that Isabella (1990) terms *aftermath*. During the aftermath period, the changes are evaluated and interpreted, conclusions are drawn about the new organisation's strengths and weaknesses, and winners and losers are identified. The new order is then established in people's minds.

## Evaluation

This framework draws upon a social psychological paradigm to understand how culture change is initiated and the behavioural and cognitive experiences of those involved. It pays attention to the ritualised behaviour associated with organisational change, and it usefully couches culture change as a problem of adaptation to external and internal environments. It is widely applicable to any type of organisation and to any level within an organisation. However, the model paints a linear picture of change, and it appears to expect adaptation to occur without serious upset or bitter conflict, which is arguably not the fate of most change programmes. It does not tell the change agent what to do, being more descriptive than prescriptive. This framework does not seek to address the question of whether a change programme is advisable or successful.

# Summary of the five culture change models

Despite the obvious differences between the five models discussed above, all of these models share common foci on a *crisis* as the trigger for culture change, on the role of *leaders* to detect a need for and to shape and implement change, on *success* to consolidate the new order and counter resistance, and on *relearning* and *re-education* to explain the efficient assimilation of cultural change (*see* Box 1.5).

---

**Box 1.5**   Key ingredients of culture change

- Triggered by a perception of *crisis*
- Initiated and shaped by strong *leaders*
- Consolidated by perceived *success*
- Mediated by *relearning/re-education*

---

The models illustrate how organisational culture change can be understood in different ways. No conclusions can be drawn concerning which is the best model to apply. Collectively, the models indicate the complexity of organisational culture and organisational change. This level of difficulty is matched by the high level of unpredictability of success or failure of programmes of organisational culture change. It should be remembered that a basic function of organisational culture is to stabilise and establish a way of living. Resistance to change is therefore inherent to culture.

Arguably no model could incorporate the complexity involved in actual culture change. However, organisational change is both necessary and increasingly frequent, with all of the attendant stresses and strains caused by instability and unpredictability. Perhaps the key challenge, therefore, is to try to understand the difficulties inherent in such change and the practical implications for participants in terms of the destabilising of their whole lives. The NHS is undergoing a number of change programmes simultaneously, which can be expected to impact on its culture in both expected and unexpected ways. The way in which these changes are designed and implemented (the *process*) will probably affect the outcomes.

# How can organisational culture be assessed?

In this section we have reviewed a number of different perspectives on organisational culture, the role of organisational leadership and models of organisational culture change. The theoretical approaches covered raise a number of important points that are relevant to the assessment of organisational culture and culture change.

- Organisational culture is a contested domain.
- A number of different theoretical approaches have been used.
- Organisational culture is a multiple phenomenon – a coalition of patterns of meaning forged by human groups and subcultures.
- A health service culture is produced not only by employees, but also by patients and the public.
- The relative power of subcultures and other influences in defining a dominant culture is an important issue.
- Leadership plays an important and complex role in culture and culture change.

# Some reflections on organisational culture

We should not underestimate the level of difficulty involved in attempting to analyse any type of culture, or the pitfalls of adopting a polarised perspective. We should try to avoid two such pitfalls in particular, namely that of intellectually weak, woolly and lazy thinking (the bane of so much work on management topics) and, at the opposite pole, that of spurious operational terminology (which is so unhelpful in the social sciences). Given that the 'object' of our analysis is something as broad, complex and contested as organisational culture, it will be fruitful to adopt '*a combination of loose and strict thinking* (which) is the most precious tool of science' (Bateson, 1941). We can better grasp what Bateson had in mind when he referred to this combination of loose and strict thinking through his own experience of cultural analysis:

> I was especially interested in studying what I called the 'feel' of culture, and I was bored with the conventional study of the more formal details. I went out to New Guinea with that much vaguely clear – and in one of my first letters home I complained of the

hopelessness of putting any sort of salt on the tail of such an imponderable concept as the 'feel' of culture. I had been watching a casual group of natives chewing betel, spitting, laughing, joking, etc., and I felt acutely the tantalizing impossibility of what I wanted to do.

(Bateson, 1941)

What he actually did was to define concepts of 'ethos' and 'cultural structure'. He pictured their relationship as being like a river and its bank: 'The river molds the banks and the banks guide the river. Similarly, the ethos molds the cultural structure and is guided by it'. However, as the date for his next field trip approached, and with the final chapter of his book on the New Guinea Latmul tribe still unwritten, Bateson began to doubt his own categories. He found that any of the examples of Latmul culture that he had observed could be categorised as either ethos or cultural structure, and he feared that his analysis might turn to dust. In practice, only a revision was required to accommodate the problem. He discovered that he had fallen prey to the common fallacy of treating analytical concepts as concrete realities, when they are in fact only labels for points of view adopted by the investigator or the natives. This argument has been expressed succinctly by WJH Sprott:

> Theories are not utterances of absolute truth, they are useful devices for understanding. If a theory ceases to be useful, we cast it aside and turn to another; theories are to be *used* rather than believed in.

(Sprott, quoted in Brown, 1954, p. 153)

We can learn from this vignette that at certain points in the analysis of organisational culture it is helpful to adopt or invent metaphors suggestive of meanings, descriptions and explanations that would not arise from a different approach. At other points it is necessary to subject these loose constructions to a rigorous critique in order to validate emergent ideas and observations. This is arguably the nature of progressive research – one has an idea and runs with it for a while, but then it is necessary to pause to catch one's breath and reflect on the plausibility and coherence of the narrative created. Thus the process continues, alternating between creative and critical phases. Yet too often the running continues and the reflective pause is not taken.

# Limitations of metaphor

If we wish to say that a healthcare organisation is like a dinosaur, or a juggernaut, or that making change is like trying to run through treacle, those similes have an expressive value. They say something about the perceptions and experiences of those who participate in such enterprises. However, we shall never locate the one 'real' organisational culture, nor therefore a perfect metaphor with which to describe it. A large healthcare organisational culture is a multiple reality. The cultural approach to analysing societies is itself a horticultural metaphor. It is so broad and contested that we should beware of being seduced into a fictional or polarised view of the object of analysis. If it includes behaviour, values and hidden assumptions, we can study these without configuring them as 'culture'. Culture is a sign that tells us something about how we can approach such things. Otherwise we risk mistaking our finger for the moon, the metaphor and the rhetoric for the living organisation.

# Culture and change

The meaningful character of culture is inextricably bound up with loss and change. If life were simply rational, and organisations were merely mechanisms of service and production, then organisational change would not provoke the strong reactions that it does. Peter Marris's analysis (Marris, 1986) of bereavement as loss of meaning, and his extension of the principle to other momentous changes, including organisational development and workplace rationalisation, is pertinent here. If culture constitutes a meaningful system, then even small changes in a working culture, such as a revised role or a change of office, may provoke apparently disproportionate reactions of anger, hostility, resistance and destructive behaviour. We can make sense of these reactions in terms of how reorganisation threatens the meaning systems of those whom it affects. Then it may be understood how the loss of a few inches of space can be threatening, and how every element of the work environment has this potential. The key point here is that change usually involves a sense of loss. Reactions to change are therefore highly significant for individuals, work groups and organisations. Even a few disaffected individuals can cause great disruption, and a disaffected workforce may be a recipe for organisational disaster. Yet typically senior executives have little sense of the mood of other participants. They are often 'out of touch' with that important reality.

Whether we adopt idealist or materialist perspectives on organisational culture, culture is strongly related to the conservative impulse. We form cultures through socially mediated meaning construction to provide a stable platform (a meaningful context) upon which to conduct our lives. For this to be effective, the platform must be reasonably predictable and durable. As the relationship between meaning and the states of affairs which it interprets is indirect, and certainly more than causal, a key way of preserving the integrity of a culture is by conservation of meaning. It is this psychosocial preservation of familiar meaning to which the conservative impulse refers. Thus culture and the conservative impulse are inseparable. We try to conserve the meaning of which a culture is made.

# Tools for measuring organisational cultures

## Introduction to culture assessment

Part 2 reviews a range of methods and instruments designed to describe and assess organisational culture. Eight instruments that appear to have the best validity to assess healthcare organisational cultures (*see* Box 2.1) are examined in detail. The salient characteristics of the instruments identified are then discussed. Finally, a summary of points to address when developing a culture assessment methodology for a healthcare organisation is proposed.

---

**Box 2.1**  Eight approaches to organisational culture assessment

*Typological approaches*
1  *Competing Values Framework*
   Types: clan, hierarchy, adhocracy and market attributes: (1) dominant characteristics or values, (2) dominant style of leadership, (3) dominant style of cohesion, (4) strategic emphasis, (5) reward systems.
2  *Organisational ideologies*
   Types: (1) power orientation, (2) role orientation, (3) task orientation, (4) self-orientation.

*Dimensional approaches*
3  *Organisational Culture Inventory*
   Orientations: satisfaction, people, security, task. Dimensions (thinking styles): (1) humanistic–helpful, (2) affiliative, (3) approval, (4) conventional, (5) dependent, (6) avoidance, (7) oppositional, (8) power, (9) competitive, (10) competence/perfectionist, (11) achievement, (12) self-actualisation.
4  *Hospital Culture Questionnaire*
   Dimensions: (1) supervision, (2) the employer, (3) role significance, (4) hospital image, (5) competitiveness, (6) benefits, (7) cohesiveness, (8) workload.

---

5 *Nursing Unit Culture Assessment Tool*
   Dimensions: preferred behaviour.
6 *Practice Culture Questionnaire*
   Dimensions: attitudes to clinical governance.
7 *Mackenzie's Culture Questionnaire*
   Dimensions: (1) employee commitment, (2) attitudes to and beliefs about innovation, (3) attitudes towards change, (4) style of conflict resolution, (5) management style, (6) confidence in the leadership, (7) openness and trust, (8) teamwork and co-operation, (9) action orientation, (10) human resource orientation, (11) consumer orientation, (12) organisational direction.
8 *Core Employee Opinions Questionnaire*
   Dimensions: employees' perceptions of working environment.

We have examined whether instruments have been tested for validity and reliability, whether they have been used in healthcare contexts, and the level of culture that they tap into. Our assessments of the instruments relate to their potential to analyse organisational cultures in the NHS and in other health systems. The review is extensive but not exhaustive, as there will certainly be other approaches that we have failed to find or about which we have been unable to obtain sufficient information to include. However, we believe this review to be the most comprehensive now available.

Schein's definition of organisational culture, the most widely acknowledged in the literature, is as follows:

> the pattern of shared basic assumptions – invented, discovered or developed by a given group as it learns to cope with its problems of external adaptation and internal integration – that has worked well enough to be considered valid and, therefore, to be taught to new members as the correct way to perceive, think and feel in relation to those problems.
>
> (Schein, 1985, p. 9)

According to Schein, the essence of an organisational culture is its characteristic pattern of assumptions, of which artefacts are expressions. Espoused values may reflect deeper assumptions or superficial rationalisations. Thus instruments for assessing culture should be designed to elicit the normally unspoken assumptions which are formed through dynamic processes of work performance and socialisation, and which guide the behaviour of organisational members imperceptibly. Thus we are not interested in methods of assessing organisational structures or task performance (although we might be interested in these factors in so far as they are informed by the basic assumptions embodied in the life of an organisation). The focus is rather on a deep ecology of the organisation – on concealed forces that have in Schein's terms 'dropped out of consciousness'. It follows that the conclusion of an organisational cultural analysis would be *a statement of the key assumptions held by participants in a given organisation.* When considering the instruments actually developed to assess organisational culture, therefore, we pay close attention to which of the three main cultural levels (assumptions, values and artefacts) each of these instruments aims to illuminate.

A diverse range of tools has been developed to assess organisational culture. They span the spectrum of qualitative and quantitative techniques, ranging from ethnography (including observation, informal interviews and attending meetings) to the administration of carefully developed survey instruments designed to measure and compare the key cultural characteristics of a single organisation, or of a number of organisations.

Proponents of qualitative and quantitative research methodologies typically disagree about the validity of their preferred approaches to data collection, and the field of organisational culture studies is no exception (Ott, 1989). Schein (1985), for example, proposes a 'clinical' approach to organisational culture analysis, viewing the organisation as a client seeking outside help in order to overcome problems that it cannot tackle alone. The key reasons why Schein believes that culture surveys do not and cannot measure culture, especially its fundamental assumptions, are as follows. First, you do not know what to ask about or what questions to design. Secondly, asking individuals about a shared phenomenon is inefficient and possibly invalid. Thirdly, the things that employees complain about may not be changeable (Schein, 1999). On the other side of the debate, proponents of questionnaire instruments argue that qualitative approaches to organisational culture analysis are too costly, involve small, unrepresentative samples of participants, and are too slow for most organisations' needs (Davies *et al.*, 1993). A few researchers have combined quantitative and qualitative approaches (Siehl and Martin, 1984; Ott, 1989).

Quantitative and qualitative approaches generate fundamentally different types of evidence whose value depends on the purpose of the research that is being undertaken. For the purposes of this project, we have tried to tread a middle line by selecting for detailed review only those methods of organisational culture measurement that have a strong 'paper-and-pencil' element (i.e. the respondent is presented with standardised verbal or written instructions to complete a task in writing, draw an image, tick boxes, etc.). We excluded unstructured ethnographic methods, because the functional aim of the review was to inform the empirical phase of our research into organisational culture and performance in the NHS.

# Methodology

We began by searching the following databases for articles on organisational culture: Medline, Cinahl, King's Fund, Helmis, Dhdata. The resulting records were assessed by a member of the project team, and a shortlist of full articles was retrieved. Bibliographies of full articles were also searched and authors of articles and instruments were contacted where possible. Experts in the field were also contacted. Of 84 articles that appeared to report the development or administration of organisational culture assessment tools, 27 relevant instruments were identified. Of these, ten instruments have been administered in healthcare organisations (five of them in the UK).

Of the ten instruments administered in healthcare organisations, eight were selected for detailed description as the most likely candidates to guide our empirical research. The instruments reviewed in detail fall into one of two categories (Fletcher and Jones, 1992). They may be *typological*, in which case they define an organisational culture in terms of a limited number of types, as in the competing values framework (Cameron and Freeman, 1991) and Harrison's typology of organisational ideologies/cultures (Harrison, 1972, 1975). Alternatively, they may be *dimensional*, profiling an organisational culture against a set of continuous variables, as in the Organisational Culture Inventory (Cooke and Rousseau, 1988). These eight instruments will now be described. (The results of these studies are reported in Part 3.)

# Eight organisational culture assessment tools

## Competing values framework

The competing values framework or model (CVF) has been used to assess and compare the culture of many different types of organisation. It was developed by Cameron and Freeman (1991) to investigate the relationship between organisational culture and effectiveness in a sample of US colleges and universities. Gerowitz *et al.* (1996) applied the CVF in a comparative study of top management team cultures in hospitals located in Canada, the UK and the USA. The same author (Gerowitz, 1998) has also used the framework to assess the impact of total quality management/continuous quality improvement (TQM/CQI) on the culture and performance of top management teams in US hospitals. Shortell *et al.* (2000) used a version of the framework to assess the impact of organisational culture and TQM on a comprehensive set of endpoints of care for coronary artery bypass graft (CABG) patients.

## Development of the competing values framework

As it is grounded in the unspoken assumptions of participants, the culture of an organisation is difficult to assess objectively. Investigators have variously inferred these shared assumptions through stories, special language, artefacts and normative values exhibited by individuals and groups in organisations (Deal and Kennedy, 1982; Bate, 1984; Trice and Beyer, 1984; Ouchi and Wilkins, 1985; Schein, 1985, 1990, 1999). The nature of these assumptions has been investigated by certain psychologists who argue that 'axes of bias' (Jones, 1961) or 'psychological archetypes' (Jung, 1973) organise individuals' experience into a limited number of categories. These categories define the different frames used by individuals to organise underlying values, assumptions and interpretations. They can also be used to identify certain types of cultures in organisations, because cultures are based on those values, assumptions and interpretations (Neuman, 1955; Neuman, 1970; Jaynes, 1976; Mitroff, 1983; Cameron and Freeman, 1991).

> Simply stated, psychological archetypes serve to organize the underlying assumptions and understandings that emerge among individuals in organizations and that become labelled cultures.
>
> (Cameron and Freeman, 1991, p. 26)

Jung's model of psychological archetypes (Jung, 1923) is the best known, and has been widely used to identify personality types. The Jungian framework has also been used to analyse organisational 'personalities'. Mitroff and Kilmann (1976), for example, found that people's descriptions of organisational cultures were consistent with the Jungian typology. These categories also serve as the basis for the competing values framework of organisational culture.

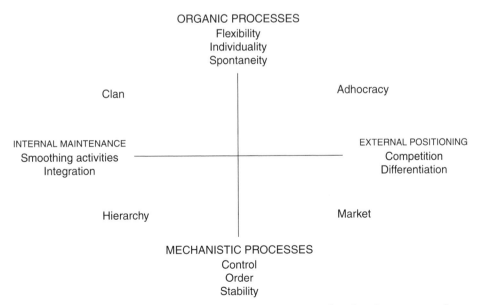

**Figure 2.1** A model of culture types for organisations (reproduced with permission from Cameron and Freeman 1991, p. 27).

The framework was constructed empirically by Quinn and Rohrbaugh (1981) through their analysis of the values held by individuals with regard to desirable organisational performance. Using a list of effectiveness criteria claimed by Campbell (1977) to be comprehensive in scope, Quinn and Rohrbaugh discovered that the criteria clustered together in a way that reproduced the Jungian framework almost exactly (Cameron and Freeman, 1991). The Jungian framework thus forms the basis of a typology of organisational cultures: 'Just as four psychological archetypes exist using the Jungian framework, so do four organizational culture types exist using the competing values model' (Cameron and Freeman, 1991, p. 27). The four culture types are *clan, hierarchy, adhocracy* and *market*.

Several authors have asserted that the strength and congruence of an organisation's culture are positively related to high levels of performance (Deal and Kennedy, 1982; Peters and Waterman, 1982; Sathe, 1983) and to smooth functioning and an absence of conflict (Quinn and McGrath, 1984). Cameron and Freeman (1991) tested these hypotheses by developing the competing values framework to examine empirically the congruence and strength of organisational cultures, in addition to their type.

Drawing on a wide literature, Cameron and Freeman (1991) identified key attributes that represent congruence of fit within each organisational culture. Congruence is defined as:

> consistency among organizational systems and components. It is congruence within a culture, rather than homogeneity among organisational subcultures or agreement among organisational respondents.
>
> (Cameron and Freeman, 1991, p. 28)

Four sets of attributes were chosen to represent the characteristics of each culture type. Box 2.2 shows the four sets of attributes together with their main characteristics.

---

**Box 2.2** A model of cultural congruence for organisations (reproduced with permission of Elsevier Science from Cameron and Freeman, 1991)

ORGANIC PROCESSES

*Type*: clan.
*Dominant attributes*: cohesiveness, participation, teamwork, sense of family.
*Leader style*: mentor, facilitator, parent figure.
*Bonding*: loyalty, tradition, interpersonal cohesion.
*Strategic emphases*: toward developing human resources, commitment, morale.

*Type*: adhocracy.
*Dominant attributes*: creativity, entrepreneurship, adaptability, dynamism.
*Leader style*: entrepreneur, innovator, risk taker.
*Bonding*: entrepreneurship, flexibility, risk.
*Strategic emphases*: toward innovation.

| | |
|---|---|
| *Type*: hierarchy.<br>*Dominant attributes*: order, rules and regulations, uniformity, efficiency.<br>*Leader style*: co-ordinator, organiser, administrator.<br>*Bonding*: rules, policies and procedures, clear expectations.<br>*Strategic emphases*: toward stability, predictability, smooth operations. | *Type*: market.<br>*Dominant attributes*: competitiveness, goal achievement, environment exchange.<br>*Leader style*: decisive, production and achievement oriented.<br>*Bonding*: goal orientation, production, competition.<br>*Strategic emphases*: toward competitive advantage and market superiority. |

The four sets of core attributes are as follows:

1  the dominant characteristics or values
2  the dominant style of leadership
3  the bases for bonding or coupling
4  the strategic emphases present in the organisation.

Cameron and Freeman administered the competing values framework to a large sample of individuals representing 334 colleges and universities in the USA. In total, 3406 individuals participated in the study (55% of the total number of individuals who received a questionnaire). The questionnaire that was mailed to each respondent contained questions assessing organisational effectiveness on the nine dimensions shown in Box 2.3.

---

**Box 2.3**  Dimensions of organisational effectiveness (reproduced with permission of Elsevier Science from Cameron and Freeman, 1991)

1  Student educational satisfaction
2  Student academic development
3  Student career development
4  Student personal development
5  Faculty and administrator employment satisfaction
6  Professional interaction
7  System openness and community interaction
8  Ability to acquire resources
9  Organisational health

---

Each of the nine dimensions of effectiveness falls into one of three domains, namely the academic domain, the morale domain and the external adaptation domain.

  Brief scenarios describe the dominant characteristics of each of the four culture types, and respondents divided 100 points between the four scenarios depending on how similar they thought each scenario was to their own organisation. This allows respondents to indicate both the type of culture(s) that characterise the organisation and the strength of the culture (i.e. the more points given, the stronger or more dominant the culture type):

> The rationale for this type of question is that the underlying assumptions related to organizational culture are more likely to emerge from questions that ask respondents to react to already constructed descriptions of organizations than from questions asking respondents to generate the descriptions themselves. ... The questions were intended as mirrors, where respondents rated the familiarity of each reflection.
>
> (Cameron and Freeman, 1991, pp. 32–3)

When respondents gave the highest number of points on each of the four questions to cultural attributes representing the same quadrant of Figure 2.1, the culture was labelled congruent. The strength of the culture was based on the number of points given to the attributes. For example, if respondents gave 70 points to an attribute, rather than 40 points, that attribute was considered to be stronger or more dominant in the culture.

It was found that no institution was characterised totally by one culture (i.e. none of them gave all 100 points to the same quadrant on all questions), but dominant cultures were clearly evident in some institutions. In total, 47 institutions (14%) were classified as having congruent cultures, whereas 32 institutions (10%) had completely incongruent cultures. Of the 47 congruent cultures, 25 (53%) were clans, 9 (19%) were adhocracies, 12 (26%) were hierarchies, and only one (2%) was a market.

Cameron and Freeman found no significant differences in organisational effectiveness between institutions with congruent cultures and those with incongruent cultures, or between those with strong cultures and those with weak cultures. However, they did find that the type of culture possessed by institutions (clan, adhocracy, hierarchy or market) showed an important association with effectiveness as well as with other organisational attributes. Clans scored highest on the four dimensions of effectiveness associated with the morale domain, which is consistent with its emphasis on participation, consensus and cohesion. Adhocracies scored highest on the two dimensions comprising external adaptation, which is consistent with the emphasis of the adhocratic type on innovation, creativity and entrepreneurship. The market culture scored highest on the ability to acquire resources, which is appropriate to its emphasis on competitive actions and achievements. The hierarchy culture did not score highest on any of the nine effectiveness dimensions.

We have dealt with Cameron and Freeman's original study in some detail because it will help us to understand how later investigators have adapted and applied the competing values framework to healthcare organisations. Cameron and Freeman found that culture *type* appeared to be more important in accounting for effectiveness than either *congruence* or *strength*. However, there is no single best type of culture:

The appropriate culture type depends on what dimensions of effectiveness are important and relevant to the organization. Researchers have found that as the characteristics of organizations changed over time, so did the criteria of effectiveness that were most important for its survival. ... This requires that managers be sensitive to the dominant culture types that exist in their organizations at various stages of the organizational life cycle, and capitalize on organizational strengths. When organizations have dominant cultures, they are high performers in domains consistent with these cultures. Managers should address these issues when embarking upon organizational change efforts.

(Cameron and Freeman, 1991, p. 53)

# Application of the competing values framework to healthcare organisations

Gerowitz *et al.* (1996) used the competing values framework to examine the role of top management team culture in hospitals in the UK, Canada and the USA. The study addressed three questions. First, do hospital management teams in the UK, Canada and the USA have different management cultures associated with differences in their political economies? Secondly, is management culture associated with differences in performance? Thirdly, is culture type an independent variable? Gerowitz *et al.* (1996) renamed Cameron and Freeman's four culture types and reversed the vertical axis defining the organic–mechanistic continuum. Table 2.1 presents Cameron and Freeman's original labels alongside those of Gerowitz and colleagues. The original labels are arguably more transparently meaningful than Gerowitz's revised versions (e.g. 'hierarchy' has face validity, whereas 'empirical' is obscure), and the reversal of one axis appears to be an arbitrary change.

Gerowitz *et al.* (1996) also renamed two of the four attributes, so that 'dominant attributes' became 'staff climate', and 'bonding' became 'reward systems'. A total of 265 hospitals were surveyed, including 100 hospitals in the UK, 45 hospitals in Ontario, Canada and 120 hospitals in the USA. The response

**Table 2.1:** Comparison of the different labels for the four competing values framework culture types

| Cameron and Freeman (1991) | Gerowitz et al. (1996) and Gerowitz (1998) | Shortell et al. (2000) |
|---|---|---|
| Clan | Clan | Group |
| Hierarchy | Empirical | Hierarchical |
| Adhocracy | Open | Developmental |
| Market | Rational | Rational |

rates were 34%, 52% and 75%, respectively. All of the hospitals that were sampled were larger than 150 beds. All of the Canadian and UK hospitals were not-for-profit institutions. Of the respondent hospitals in the USA, 80% were not-for-profit and 20% were investor-owned for-profit institutions. The top management team, defined as the Chief Executive Officer and up to seven key staff selected by the latter, completed the survey.

Proponents of TQM believe that its successful introduction produces changes in organisational culture and improvements in performance. In a further study, Gerowitz (1998) used the competing values framework to assess the impact of TQM/CQI interventions on the culture and performance of top management teams in 120 hospitals in the USA. All of the hospitals were over 150 beds in size. Questionnaires were mailed to CEOs, who were asked if they had initiated formal TQM efforts. Institutions that replied in the affirmative were classed as TQM initiators. Those that had not engaged in formal TQM were classed as non-initiators. In addition to completing the questionnaire personally, each CEO was asked to give the questionnaire to each member of his or her top management team. Because organisational size had been shown to influence hospital performance, size and sponsorship were selected as controls. A total of 271 complete responses were received from 52 not-for-profit hospitals (a response rate of 43%).

In a prospective cohort study, Shortell et al. (2000) assessed the impact of TQM and organisational culture on a comprehensive set of endpoints of care for CABG patients, including risk-adjusted adverse outcomes, clinical efficiency, patient satisfaction, functional health status and cost of care. A total of 3045 eligible patients from 16 hospitals were involved in the study. At each of the 16 hospitals, an average of 54 clinicians and administrative support staff directly involved in the care of CABG patients completed a two-part questionnaire designed to assess the hospital's TQM implementation and culture. An overall response rate of 55% was achieved. The organisational culture section of the questionnaire (Gillies et al., 1992) used a 20-item instrument based on the competing values framework. Once again the names of the culture types were changed, although their identity remained vertually the same. *Group cultures* emphasise affiliation, teamwork, co-ordination and participation, *developmental cultures* emphasise risk taking, innovation and change, *rational cultures* emphasise efficiency and achievement, and *hierarchical cultures* emphasise rules, regulations and reporting relationships. Shortell et al. (2000) postulated that patients would experience more positive clinical outcomes, greater clinical efficiency, higher functional health status, higher patient satisfaction and lower costs as the extent to which the hospitals had implemented TQM and had a supportive (i.e. group) culture increased.

The internal consistency reliability coefficient (Cronbach's alpha) for the group culture scale was 0.79. Analysis of variance (ANOVA) tests verified that individual responses to the culture instrument could be validly aggregated at the hospital level, as the within-hospital variability of responses was less than the between-hospital variability. The $F$-value was 8.97 for the group culture measure ($P \leqslant 0.0001$).

The competing values framework purports to elicit tacit assumptions underlying an organisation's culture by invoking a typology of Jungian archetypes. It has good face validity and acceptable internal consistency. However, it is questionable whether four culture types are sufficient to categorise the diversity of organisational forms and types that actually exist. It is also questionable whether the framework actually goes any deeper than employees' opinions of their workplace, managers, formality/informality, rewards systems, and so on. As Schein (1999) argues, these are important dimensions of the hospital's climate, and so they should be measured. However, it is likely that the hospital culture's tacit assumptions remain unarticulated. For example are there any hidden assumptions concerning the likelihood of successful treatment outcomes according to the patient's age, ethnicity or gender? Would this affect what type of information and recommendation was given to patients? If they do not get to the all-important level of assumptions, Schein may be correct in maintaining that surveys only address espoused values concerning working relationships.

# The Organisational Culture Inventory

The Organisational Culture Inventory (OCI) has been used in most economic sectors. Studies using the OCI in healthcare organisations include evaluations by McDaniel and Stumpf (1993) and Seago (1997) of the cultures of acute care hospitals, an examination by Ingersoll et al. (2000) of the relationships between organisational culture, commitment and readiness to change, and an assessment by Seago (1996) of nursing unit culture. Shortell et al. (1994) and Zimmerman et al. (1991) have used a revised version of the OCI in the National ICU Study to examine caregiver interaction.

The theory behind the OCI is that culture is composed of the shared cognitions of a social group acquired through socialisation processes and exposure to a variety of culture-bearing elements (Geertz, 1973; Smircich, 1983; Cooke and Rousseau, 1988). These elements include observable activities and behaviour, communicated information, and artefacts produced by the group's task-related and social interaction. Culture-based cognitions form part of the 'enacted environment' (Weick, 1979a). Individuals organise their experience of the world in order to manage its inherent uncertainty by constructing meaning for events. This process of meaning construction is a collective enterprise that operates in parallel to the instrumental function of the organisation. In an organisational culture the process of social construction tends to focus thinking and behaviour towards those behaviours that are generally expected and rewarded by the organisation. This process can lead to the formation and maintenance of a cohesive dominant culture, but also to the formation of a differentiated culture or a set of subcultures. Among other differences, subcultures typically reflect differences in the main occupational groups that make up the workforce of an organisation. In addition, countercultures sometimes arise that conflict with other subcultures or with the dominant culture (Martin and Seihl, 1983).

A culture can be said to have two key tendencies that are relevant to its assessment, namely direction and intensity (Trice and Beyer, 1984; Cooke and Rousseau, 1988). Direction relates to the substance of the culture, including its artefacts, behaviour patterns, values, shared cognitions and basic assumptions. Intensity relates to the degree of consensus about the culture among unit members, and to the strength of connections between expectations, behaviour and rewards.

The OCI (Cooke and Lafferty, 1987) was designed as part of a diagnostic system for individual change and organisational development, and is the property of the Human Synergistics company. It is linked to the Life Styles Inventory (Lafferty, 1973), which measures the self-perceptions of individuals with regard to 12 'thinking styles' that are claimed to be causally related to such outcomes as managerial effectiveness, quality of interpersonal relationships and individual well-being:

> Based on these 12 styles, the culture inventory assesses the ways in which organizational members are *expected* to think and behave in relation to their tasks and to other people.
> (Cooke and Rousseau, 1988, p. 252)

Respondents to the OCI answer 120 questions describing behaviours or personal styles that might be expected of members of their organisation (e.g. 'compete rather than co-operate'). The 12 styles are as follows: (1) humanistic–encouraging; (2) affiliative; (3) approval; (4) conventional; (5) dependent; (6) avoidance; (7) oppositional; (8) power; (9) competitive; (10) competence/perfectionist; (11) achievement; (12) self-actualising.

Although the 12 thinking styles were developed to reflect the thinking and behavioural tendencies of individuals, qualitative and quantitative evidence has been advanced by Cooke and Rousseau (1988) to suggest that they also reflect 'the direction or content of certain organizational norms and expectations' (Cooke and Rousseau, 1988, p. 252). Thus the OCI is intended to measure the content and strength of organisational norms and expectations. It achieves this by helping respondents to clarify their own experiences of their organisation's culture relative to the 12 thinking styles, by comparison with the aggregate perceptions of colleagues, and to understand how their own styles might be affected by organisational norms (Cooke and Rousseau, 1988).

# The development of the OCI

The OCI has been applied to a wide range of organisations, including manu-facturing and high-technology firms, research and development laboratories, educational institutions, Government agencies and volunteer organisations. In the course of its development, 20 000 individuals in more than 100 organi-sations completed the OCI (Cooke and Rousseau, 1988). It contains 120 items, producing 12 scales of 10 items each. Each item describes a behaviour or style that might be expected of participants in an organisation. On a scale of 1 to 5, respondents indicate the extent to which each behaviour helps people to 'fit in' and 'meet expectations' in their organisation.

The Cronbach alpha reliability coefficients for the 12 scales are based on data from 661 respondents (526 members of 18 organisations using the OCI for organisational development, and 135 participants in executive development programmes or graduate business programmes) (Cooke and Rousseau, 1988). Internal consistency scores for the subscales range from 0.67 to 0.92. The results of a principal-components factor analysis of the OCI indicate that three empir-ical factors underlie the 12 scales:

1 *people/security culture*, with norms and expectations for *approval, conventional, dependent* and *avoidance* styles
2 *satisfaction culture*, with norms and expectations for *achievement, self-actualisa-tion, humanistic–encouraging* and *affiliative* styles
3 *task/security culture*, with norms and expectations for *oppositional, power, competitive* and *competence/perfectionist* styles.

The analysis-of-variance data (Cooke and Rousseau, 1988, p. 261, table 6) show intra-organisational consensus with regard to perceived norms and expectations, although the level of agreement varies across culture styles.

Thomas *et al.* (1990) report that the OCI has been used in various healthcare organisations. Their own study of a metropolitan community hospital in the USA used the OCI to measure nursing culture. In total, 56 out of 225 nurses at the hospital completed the inventory. The Results profile in Figure 2.2 repre-sents the 'ideal' nursing culture as described by 26 registered nurses across several hospitals.

The 'ideal' nursing culture aspires to maximise organisational performance, quality of care, and individual motivation and satisfaction. The culture described is *constructive*, emphasising members' higher-order or satisfaction needs, and would promote *achievement, self-actualising, humanistic* and *affiliative* behaviours by nurses (Thomas *et al.*, 1990). The culture would minimise *passive/defensive* and *aggressive/defensive* behaviours, associated with lower-order or security needs. This ideal profile is generally consistent with the ideal profiles described by members of various for-profit organisations in manufacturing and service sectors

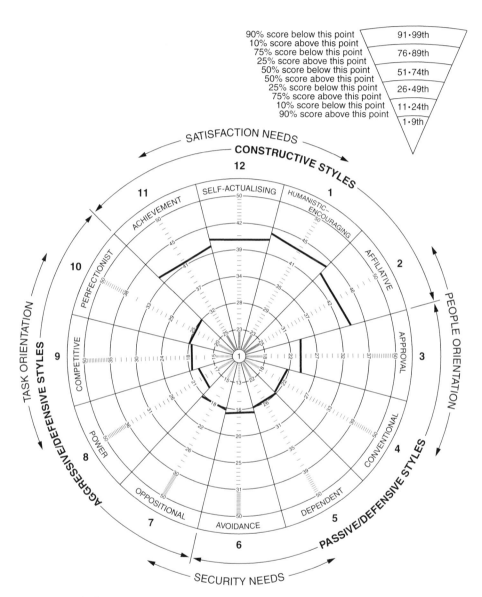

**Figure 2.2** Ideal nursing culture profile (*n* = 26 registered nurses). Cooke and Lafferty, 1987; copyright 1989 by Human Synergistics, Inc. Reproduced by permission.

(cf. Cooke and Rousseau, 1988). It provides a 'benchmark' against which Thomas *et al.* (1990) compared actual nursing culture profiles. Figure 2.3 shows the actual culture profile of staff nurses compared with administrators.

Figure 2.3 shows that the overall nursing culture at this hospital is weak. Nursing personnel (denoted by solid lines) do not report strong norms and expectations for any of the 12 cultural styles. The level of agreement among nurses with regard to these norms and expectations is also low, further indicating a weak culture. In addition, slight differences are evident between sub-groups. The administrators report slightly higher expectations for satisfaction-orientated behaviours such as *achievement* and *self-actualisation* (Thomas *et al.*, 1990, p. 20).

This example illustrates how the OCI can be used to assess and compare organisational cultures, subcultures and even countercultures in healthcare organisations. Alternative assessments could compare nursing, medical, management and other subcultures within and between healthcare organisations.

Ingersoll *et al.* (2000) applied the OCI in a study that was undertaken to determine the relationships between organisational culture, organisational commitment and organisational readiness in a sample of employees participating in a hospital-wide redesign process. The study setting consisted of two tertiary-care hospitals in the USA, which were in the process of a patient-focused redesign programme. The sample consisted of all employees involved in the redesign process. All nursing, administrative and ancillary support personnel were included. Of a total of 2157 questionnaires that were distributed, 887 (41.1%) were returned, of which 684 (31.7% of the total) were usable. Due to funding limitations, copies of the OCI were sent to a random 25% sample of the study population. The specific response rate for the OCI was not reported. The internal consistency coefficient alpha scores for the OCI ranged from 0.79 to 0.96. Organisational commitment was measured by the Commitment/Energy subscale of the Pasmore Sociotechnical Systems Assessment Survey (Pasmore, 1988). Organisational readiness was measured by the Innovativeness and Co-operation subscales of the Sociotechnical Systems Assessment Survey (STSAS) (Pasmore, 1988).

Ingersoll *et al.* (2000) conceive of culture, commitment and readiness as different but related variables. However, it is worth considering commitment and readiness as potential components of culture. Organisational commitment is defined as an individual's identification with and involvement in a particular organisation. It is characterised by a strong belief in and acceptance of the organisation's goals and values, a willingness to exert considerable effort on behalf of the organisation, and a strong desire to maintain membership of the organisation (Porter *et al.*, 1974; Moday *et al.*, 1979; Ingersoll *et al.*, 2000). It is plausible that an individual's level of commitment could form an assumption that affects their behaviour. For instance, if the individual anticipated a long-term career in a healthcare organisation, they might behave in a different way to that displayed

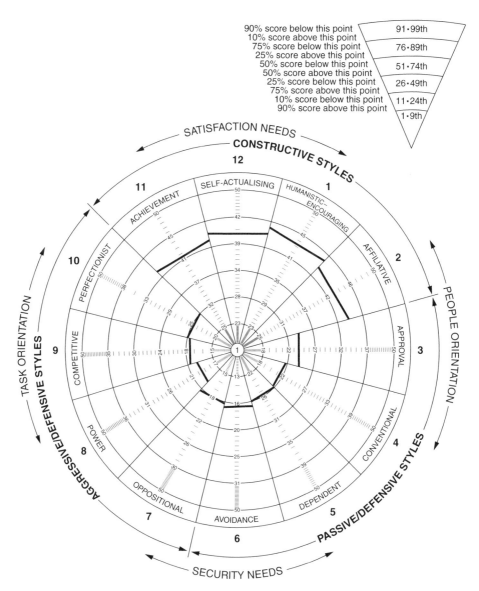

**Figure 2.3** Culture profile: staff nurses vs. nursing administrators. Cooke and Lafferty, 1987; copyright 1989 by Human Synergistics, Inc. Reproduced by permission.

if only a brief stay in the organisation was expected. Retention of nursing staff has become a key personnel challenge in recent years in both the UK and the USA. Chronic high vacancy levels and high rates of turnover are unlikely to support improvements in the quality of care. If organisational commitment was found to be in decline, one might expect levels of commitment to the quality and efficiency of care to decline as well. Studies of organisational commitment, which have focused mainly on the relationship with staff turnover, have found that employee commitment is positively correlated with job involvement and number of years in the organisation, and negatively correlated with work overload and turnover (Moday *et al.*, 1979; Arnold and Feldman, 1982; Michaels and Spector, 1982; Rusbult and Farrell, 1983; Reilly and Orsak, 1991). From a human resources perspective, therefore, organisational commitment could form an important component of organisational culture. If this was so, an assessment of healthcare organisational culture should consider including organisational commitment as one dimension relating to the recruitment and retention of staff, and to the quality and efficiency of the services that are delivered.

Organisational commitment is also relevant to current policy proposals to devolve autonomy of decision making in the NHS. It would be risky to increase autonomy of frontline staff without an assessment of their commitment to the organisation and its goals. High levels of autonomy combined with low levels of commitment might lead to a proliferation of activities (including job seeking) that ignore or conflict with the organisation's 'core values' or 'mission'.

Similar arguments apply to organisational readiness, which refers to the impact of previous experience of organisational change on further organisational change initiatives. It has been suggested that previous experience of organisational change increases the likelihood of favourable redesign outcomes, because employees have learned to be more adaptable (Ingersoll *et al.*, 2000). However, no empirical evidence for this assertion is given. Might not previous organisational changes tend to deter employees from embracing further change efforts? An assessment of organisational culture could usefully attempt to gauge readiness to change if one purpose of assessing organisational culture is to inform future strategies for change. Resistance to change could be an integral part of organisational culture.

McDaniel and Stumpf (1993) used the OCI to evaluate the culture of seven acute-care hospitals using a random sample of 209 subjects. This study reported a Cronbach's alpha value of 0.90 for individual-level data and acceptable (*sic*) construct and content validity (Seago, 1997). Seago (1995) performed a principal-component factor analysis on the individual-level data from her study and generated the same three empirical factors as Cooke and Lafferty (1987) and Cooke and Rousseau (1988).

A common issue for instruments such as the OCI relates to the aggregation of individual scores to represent a collective phenomenon such as organisational culture. If the study question relates to a group variable, then surely the unit of analysis should be the group, not the individual (Seago, 1997). In most of the studies that were conducted using the OCI, the individual was used as the unit of analysis (Thomas *et al.*, 1990; McDaniel and Stumpf, 1993; McDaniel, 1995) but the culture data were reported as a group finding (Seago, 1997). Seago (1996) used the nursing unit as the unit of analysis and used the group means as the group culture score, but did not evaluate the reliability or validity of the OCI using aggregated data. Only Shortell *et al.* (1994) have reported group-level data and evaluated the aggregated data for appropriateness.

# Harrison's Organisation Ideology Questionnaire

Harrison (1972) has identified four organisational ideologies, namely *power, role, task* and *person*. His definition of ideology − 'a commonly held set of doctrines, myths and symbols' (Harrison, 1975, p. 103) − makes it practically synonymous with culture. Harrison developed the questionnaire to promote discussions about organisation ideology using the conceptual framework presented in his original article (Harrison, 1972, 1975). No norms have been collected for the instrument, nor has its validity or reliability been assessed. Even so, Harrison's fourfold typology appears to have good face validity, and is widely cited and used in the literature on organisational culture (Ott, 1989; Litwinenko and Cooper, 1994).* The inclusion of the questionnaire in the *1975 Annual Handbook for Group Facilitators* (Jones and Pfeiffer, 1975) has led to its application to a wide variety of individuals and organisations. The only reported application of Harrison's typology to a healthcare organisation is in Litwinenko and Cooper's study of the impact of trust status on the culture of a health authority (Litwinenko and Cooper, 1994).

## *The development of Harrison's typology*

Harrison first presented his ideological analysis of organisations in a brief but influential essay published in the *Harvard Business Review* in 1972. Thus:

> While the term 'organization ideologies' is perhaps unfortunately ambiguous, it is the best name I can apply to the systems of thought that are central determinants of the character of organizations. An organization's ideology affects the behavior of its people, its ability

---

* Handy (1995) acknowledges Harrison as the source of his typology of Greek gods to symbolise organisational culture. Handy slightly modified Harrison's instrument and named it *Questionnaire on the Cultures of Organisations.*

to effectively meet their needs and demands, and the way it copes with its external environment. Furthermore, much of the conflict that surrounds organization change is really ideological struggle.

(Harrison, 1972, p. 119)

We can substitute culture for ideology without any loss of meaning. Harrison views the functions performed by organisation ideology/culture as follows:

- specifying the goals and values towards which the organisation should be directed and by which its performance should be measured
- prescribing appropriate relationships between individuals and the organisation (i.e. the psychological or social 'contract' that determines what the organisation can expect from its personnel, and vice versa)
- indicating what types of control and the extent of control that should be exerted over behaviour
- depicting which qualities and characteristics of organisational members should be valued and rewarded (or punished)
- showing members how to treat one another – competitively or co-operatively, honestly or dishonestly, closely or distantly
- establishing appropriate methods of coping with the external environment – aggressive exploitation, responsible negotiation, proactive exploration.

Harrison's conceptual framework (Harrison, 1972) postulates four organisational ideological/cultural orientations, namely *power orientation, role orientation, task orientation* and *person orientation*.

## Power-oriented culture

A power-oriented culture tries to dominate its environment and defeat all competition. Those who are powerful try to exert absolute control over subordinates. The law of the jungle prevails among executives, who fight for personal advantage against their peers. A power culture is jealous of its territory and expansionist in outlook. It strives to expand its sphere of control at others' expense, often exploiting other weaker organisations. In addition to this savage–imperialist form, there is also a paternalistic form of power orientation, especially among old-established family-owned firms. The senior members of such firms also attach a high value to 'face' and abide by a code of honour in their dealings with their peers.

> This is the power orientation in a velvet glove. But when the benevolent authority is crossed or challenged, from either within or without, the iron fist is very likely to appear again. In such cases, the test of power orientation is how hard a person or organization will fight for power and position when these are at issue.
>
> (Harrison, 1972, p. 121)

Arguably the power orientation is evident in the NHS in some of the attitudes, values and assumptions that are evinced by the medical profession. Medicine is a pre-entry qualification occupation that is controlled by a single 'union' (the British Medical Association). This allows a high degree of control over who enters the profession (conducive to nepotism), their professional education and training, their standards of professional conduct, the demarcation of their specialties within the profession, and a protectionist attitude towards the work of the profession as a whole. Although it traditionally exhibits a paternalistic power orientation, the introduction of general management in the NHS may have stung the medical profession into a more aggressive stance, as witnessed for example by the British Medical Association's threat to organise a mass withdrawal of family general practitioners from the NHS.* Although governments in the 1990s introduced a number of strategies to try to weaken the power base of NHS doctors, these have all largely failed, and arguably they will continue to fail for as long as medicine in the UK remains an autonomous, 'self-policing' profession.

## Role-oriented culture

A role-oriented culture values rationality and orderliness. Competition and conflict are regulated by rules and procedures. Rights and privileges are tightly defined and adhered to. Predictability, respectability and stability are valued as highly as competence, such that the correct response tends to be more highly valued than the effective one. Although most commercial organisations cannot afford the extreme rigidity of a pure role orientation, certain sectors where control over the market is high (e.g. banking, public utilities, educational institutions and some Civil Service departments) have traditionally exhibited a strong role orientation. It is plausible that the NHS exhibits a strong role orientation connected with its historical demarcation of roles and hierarchy of occupational groups, and its near monopolistic control over the healthcare market. Privatisation and competition have eroded this type, although even in some privatised utilities its vestigial attitudes and values may be encountered.

## Task-oriented culture

The task-oriented culture values goal achievement above all else:

> The goal need not be economic; it could be winning a war, converting the heathen, reforming a government, or helping the poor. The important thing is that the organization's structure, functions and activities are all evaluated in terms of their contribution to the superordinate goal.
>
> (Harrison, 1972, p. 122)

---

*Beecham L (2001) *BMJ*. **322**: 1381.

Flexibility is key to the task-oriented culture, and nothing is allowed to obstruct the accomplishment of the task. If established authority structures, systems or procedures impede progress towards the superordinate goal, they are swept aside and replaced. Individual interests are subsumed to the organisation's objectives such that those who lack the necessary knowledge and skills are regarded as dispensable. The emphasis is on a rapid response to changing conditions. Alliances and collaborations are formed on the basis of mutual goals and interests. Examples of organisations with task-oriented cultures might include leading-edge high-technology firms, internet.com companies and other high-risk enterprises that operate in fast-moving, unstable markets. A task orientation appears to be largely absent from the NHS culture, mainly because the relationships between demand and supply remain relatively stable and predictable.

## Person-oriented culture

The person-oriented culture reverses the basic priority of the other three types in that its primary function is to serve the needs of its members. Whereas some organisations evaluate the worth of individual members as tools, and accept or reject them accordingly, person-oriented organisations are evaluated as tools by their members. Authority in person-oriented organisations is kept to a minimum. Instead, individuals are expected to influence each other through example, helpfulness and caring.

Consensus methods of decision making are the norm, and individuals are not usually expected to do things that conflict with their personal preferences and values. Examples of people-oriented organisations might include groups of professionals who have joined together for research and development, and some consulting firms. Person-oriented firms are generally not very interested in growth or profit maximisation. They are more likely to operate in order to make enough money to provide their members with a comfortable living and opportunities to do meaningful and enjoyable work with congenial people.

A person-oriented culture is not obvious in the NHS.

Harrison maintains that an organisation's ideology/culture orientation profoundly affects its performance by determining how decisions are made, how human resources are used, and how the external environment is dealt with. He also points to a basic tension running through the four cultural types, which is the conflict between the values and attributes that advance the interests of people on the one hand, and the values and attributes that advance the interests of the organisation on the other. For most organisations there will be no perfect fit with any of the four culture types. Indeed, organisations may be composed of several parts, each emphasising a different culture type, which increases the potential for conflict due to different values and outlooks.

> For example, instead of one 'company spirit' there will be several 'company spirits', all different and very likely antagonistic. In this environment ... one can imagine, in fact, that the most important job of top management will not be directing the business but, instead, managing the integration of its parts.
>
> (Harrison, 1972, p. 128)

One may imagine that organisations such as the NHS and other health systems, with their collection of sharply differentiated occupational cultures, could well be inhabited by a plurality of 'company spirits'. Whether this is so, whether these spirits are antagonistic, and whether there is a need for their closer integration are all questions that could usefully be answered by empirical research using Harrison's typology.

Harrison's culture questionnaire (Harrison, 1975) consists of 20 items. For each item, respondents are asked to rank four statements in terms of (1) their organisation's existing culture and (2) their own preferred organisational culture. The two sets of responses are then compared. For each culture type, the number of individuals in the group of respondents who gave their lowest score (sum of ranks) to that ideology is recorded. This gives an indication of the convergence or divergence of values within the group, and the extent to which the group's values as a whole conflict with those of the organisation. In his questionnaire, Harrison (1975) renamed the person-oriented culture as 'self-orientation'.

Litwinenko and Cooper (1994) used Harrison's typology to examine the effects of radical changes in the NHS, in particular the adoption of trust status by one health authority. A longitudinal design, incorporating pre- and post-trust measures, was adopted in order to study the effects of trust status on perceived organisational culture and the effects over time. Questionnaires based on Harrison's original were sent out one month prior to the health authority achieving trust status, and again 12 months after the adoption of trust status.

A 30% random sample was taken from each occupational group. Out of a total of 1050 questionnaires that were sent out, 539 were returned completed, yielding a response rate of 51.3%. At the second survey point, out of a total of 539 questionnaires that were sent out, 273 were returned completed, giving a response rate of 50.6%.

Litwinenko and Cooper relabelled Harrison's person/self-orientation as 'support culture'. Their questionnaire consisted of 16 statements that respondents were required to rate on a six-point scale ranging from 'very strongly agree' to 'very strongly disagree'. Quantitative data from the questionnaire were triangulated with data obtained from anonymous exit questionnaires routinely given to staff leaving trust employment voluntarily. In addition to asking leavers why they had left and their destination, their perceptions of the organisation's culture using Harrison's typology were addressed.

Following Harrison, Litwinenko and Cooper predicted that the trust would be unlikely to be characterised predominantly by one cultural type. An NHS trust contains occupational subgroups whose cultures are shaped by their differing functions, roles and internal divisions. Therefore Litwinenko and Cooper (1994) analysed their data in terms of the sample as a whole, occupational grouping, and clinical or non-clinical contact.

Ott (1989) administered Harrison's questionnaire to the staff of one company, and his observations of the process highlight some of its strengths and limitations in a useful manner. A significant number of respondents volunteered the information that completing the questionnaire had caused them personal discomfort because it required them to think about aspects of their organisational life that they normally suppressed. The questions made them consciously recognise how their 'silly' behaviours were connected with generally held beliefs in the firm:

> Many of the Jones & Jones assumptions had been forgotten or suppressed. Some of them are not very noble. Yet these people continue to live in the culture, transmitting it to newcomers. Moreover, whereas behaviors can be modified, ideologies have an aura of permanence − just like any other accepted truths.
>
> (Ott, 1989, p. 119)

Although Ott (1989) found scores on Harrison's four orientations revealing, the real value of the questionnaire was that completing it made people realise their basic cultural assumptions, which in turn made his other data collection activities much more fruitful. However, this strength also posed a methodological problem, as the administration of the instrument tended to bias all of Ott's subsequent data collection. The instrument was often referred to by respondents in interviews and discussions. Ott's conclusion raises an important and paradoxical distinction which underlies the literature on organisational culture, but is rarely articulated:

> Should Harrison's instrument be used as a proxy indicator or to get directional clues about organizational culture? In a study conducted for academic purposes, no, I don't believe so. Its effect on data collected through other methods seems to have been great. On the other hand, in a study initiated by an organization's request for help, I would not hesitate to use it again. The advantages far outweigh the potential problems of interaction contamination.
>
> (Ott, 1989, p. 119)

Two questions are raised by that passage − first, whether a study is conducted for theoretical or practical purposes, and secondly, whether it is possible to measure without intervening in what is being measured. Schein (1985, 1999) makes a similar distinction to the first point when he remarks on the differences between the aims of anthropological and clinical approaches to organisational culture. The second question raises Heisenberg's 'uncertainty principle' (Heisenberg, 1958), which some scholars have invoked in order to relate social theory to theoretical physics. Translated into organisational terms, the uncertainty principle refers to the apparent impossibility of measuring a phenomenon (e.g. the velocity of a subatomic particle, or a person's perception of an organisation's culture) without simultaneously altering what is being measured (i.e. the particle's trajectory, or the criteria by which a culture is perceived and assessed). In practice, what the uncertainty principle tells us is that we can never be quite certain what it is that we are measuring — the 'natural' perception of the culture, or perceptions of culture that are artificially induced by the instrument.

Perhaps the 'solution' to both of these questions is the same — we must discard the idea that measuring organisational culture is an analytical science in the logical-positivistic sense, and instead embrace a more pragmatic and constructivist approach to the question. Such an approach acknowledges that any measurement of culture involves the collective construction of a narrative about the organisation, and this narrative will be assimilated into and may possibly change the culture. This narrative tells a story about life in the organisation that participants can identify with and endorse. A year later, the story might be reconstructed and different events and details might be emphasised. A description of an organisation's culture should therefore aim to reflect the culture itself. If the culture is pluralistic, being composed of many subcultural narratives, then the description should not attempt to add a unifying gloss to distort that plurality. Thus we would not expect to find statements such as 'NHS culture is this or that type', but rather we would expect to find statements such as 'NHS culture is this type, and this type, and this type, and . . .', together with qualifying statements relating to who perceives the culture to be of certain types, and in what proportions.

Another limitation of Harrison's typology is that, like the competing values framework, it invokes only four cultural types. This inevitably imposes restrictions on the variety of perceptions of cultural plurality.

# The Hospital Culture Questionnaire

Sieveking *et al.* (1993) developed an unnamed hospital employee opinion questionnaire that was designed to measure hospital culture from the employee's viewpoint. For convenience, we term this instrument the Hospital Culture Questionnaire (HCQ).

In 1987 and 1989, Sieveking *et al.* (1993) administered the HCQ in group settings to all employees of private hospitals owned by a for-profit company (HCA UK Ltd). The facilities ranged from 32 to 100 beds and were located in 10 cities in the UK. The total number of participants in 1987 was 578 (60% of all employees), and the total number in 1989 was 771 (75%). In 1987, 337 of the respondents had direct clinical responsibilities (medical/paramedical services, nursing, operating theatre, outpatients/health screening and auxiliary screening) and 241 respondents had non-clinical responsibilities (administration, food, services and housekeeping/laundry). In 1989, the corresponding numbers were 435 and 336, respectively.

# The development of the Hospital Culture Questionnaire

Sieveking's survey was intended to generate information to help corporate and hospital managers to gauge employee sentiment, so that they could develop concrete management plans for human resource and quality improvement issues. Initially, an 86-item questionnaire was constructed with responses on a 5-point scale ranging from 'strongly agree' to 'strongly disagree'. There was also an 'I don't know' option.

The questions addressed the following areas:

- perceived quality of care
- institutional atmosphere
- supervision
- fairness of employment practices
- staffing and workloads
- teamwork
- the role significance of individual workers
- communications
- general morale
- pay and benefits
- relationships with consultants
- the corporation as employer
- the concept of private for-profit healthcare.

In order to determine the internal consistency of the instrument, data from 1987 and 1989 were submitted separately to factor analysis (principal components analysis with varimax rotation and pairwise deletion). Scales of employee opinion were derived by grouping together individual items with a factor loading on the same factor of at least 0.50, in 1987 and 1989 separately. Items that did not load to that degree were not included on any scale.

The factor analysis resulted in eight scales, which included 50 of the original 86 items. Thus the HCQ measures the following eight empirical factors:

1 supervision
2 the employer
3 role significance

4 hospital image
5 competitiveness
6 benefits
7 cohesiveness
8 workload.

Coefficient alpha scores for the eight factors ranged from 0.61 to 0.93.

Two other aspects of the study contribute to the reliability of the results for representing the structure of hospital employees' opinions. First, the study was conducted in ten hospitals, albeit in a restricted area of the hospital sector, allowing comparison between study sites. Secondly, the survey was repeated in each hospital after a two-year interval.

It is not known how the cultures of UK private health services as opposed to NHS services (or health services in private or public sectors in other countries) differ in terms of their culture and/or performance. Therefore the ability of the HCQ to assess NHS culture remains an empirical question. However, an instrument that is validated on a UK private for-profit health-worker population could be at least as useful as an instrument validated in the USA. In the context of proposals to tackle shortfalls in the supply of NHS care by contracting more patients out to the private sector, the culture and performance of private for-profit facilities should be of intrinsic interest to NHS managers, clinicians and policy makers.

Relationships between the HCQ scales were also assessed. Scores were developed for each scale by summing the percentage of respondents who 'agreed' or 'strongly agreed' with each of its items. The resulting scale scores were then intercorrelated. The correlations were found to be almost identical for clinical and non-clinical staff. Although all correlations above 0.10 were statistically significant at $P < 0.001$, they were relatively small. This indicates that the scales assessed mainly independent components of hospital culture. Thus learning how an employee feels about one factor tells us little about how he or she feels about the other seven factors. This is interesting because it tends to contradict the assumptions and findings of other studies, using different instruments, that organisational cultures can be analysed as cohesive types (Harrison, 1972, 1975; Cameron and Freeman, 1991; Shortell et al., 2000). The employees in the HCQ study tended 'not to generalise about their work experience. Rather, they make ongoing discrete evaluations of its differing facets' (Sieveking et al., 1993, p. 136). One reason for this could be that, for this study population, no overall organisational culture was perceived. Another possible explanation is that the investigators failed to differentiate between the data from the different occupational groups surveyed, as did Litwinenko and Cooper (1994) in their study. If the study population was composed of a number of occupation-based subcultures, then a clear pattern of correlations across the subcultures might not be expected.

The study is also limited to the adequacy of the 86-item pool in sampling the domain of topics that were important to employees (i.e. if a topic was not tapped by one of the 86 items, it could not appear in the final scales). The deleted individual items may well represent topics that were important to hospital employees and managers, but because they did not meet factor analytical criteria established for inclusion as elements in reliable patterns of opinion, they were excluded from the instrument (Sieveking *et al.*, 1993). This limitation is shared by all survey instruments.

# The Nursing Unit Culture Assessment Tool

The Nursing Unit Culture Assessment Tool (NUCAT) was developed by Coeling and Simms (1993), and has been utilised by Rizzo *et al.* (1994) and Goodridge and Hack (1996). It assesses 50 different behaviours, which the developers have found to be valid indicators of behaviours that are important to practising nurses and that differ between nursing units. The NUCAT is scored on a 6-point scale. It is supposed to give a comprehensive description of nursing-unit culture based on a mean unit score for each of the 50 different behaviours. Like the HCQ, all the items of the NUCAT are independent of each other, thus allowing the assessment of the unique cultural configuration of a nursing unit. The NUCAT describes a group norm for each behaviour and the degree of variation within the group, which provides an indication of the relative strength of behaviours. In addition, the NUCAT describes the respondents'/unit's preferences for the 50 behaviours. The aim is to provide the unit manager and staff with a map of their current culture and the extent of their desire to change each behaviour. This assessment of the cultural configuration, strength and preferences for change is designed to enable managers to predict whether the current culture will embrace or resist a given innovation.

Coeling and Simms (1993) developed the NUCAT and established its validity through a series of qualitative and quantitative studies that were conducted over a six-year period. A three-month participant-observational study identified relevant cultural behaviours. An open-ended questionnaire was then completed by 26 graduate nursing management students in order to fine-tune the list of variables. An initial survey instrument was then completed by 62 staff nurses in order to validate the cultural variables that were most likely to differ from one unit to another. The tool was pre-tested for reliability and validity, but no metrics were reported.

Rizzo *et al.* (1994) used the NUCAT-2 in the process of implementing a new nursing model in one hospital in the USA. A total of 235 (75%) nursing department staff members from 13 different units completed the questionnaire using a 4-point scale (where 1 = 'not at all', 2 = 'slightly', 3 = 'quite' and 4 = 'extremely'). Goodridge and Hack (1996) also used the NUCAT-2 as part of a quality improvement initiative in a 320-bed long-term care facility in Canada. Questionnaires were distributed to all 320 staff, and 170 questionnaires (53%) were returned completed. Per-unit responses ranged from 19% to 78%.

In consultation with the instrument's developers (Coeling and Simms), Rizzo *et al.* (1994) interpreted mean scores for behavioural variables of < 2.3 or > 2.7 as behaviours that were important to a unit. However, Goodridge and Hack (1996) found that these cut-off points lacked sensitivity and were not useful for discriminating between important and unimportant behaviours for their respondents. They also found that a lack of subscale development made interpretation of the results difficult:

> NUCAT-2 does allow for the identification of most preferred and least preferred discrete behaviors, but neither extreme makes explicit the broader values that underpin those behaviors nor suggests any analysis for examining the meaning of each behavior in a larger context.
>
> (Goodridge and Hack, 1996, p. 46)

Goodridge and Hack (1996) also criticised the NUCAT-2 on the grounds that it related quite directly to facility policies (e.g. whether one should call in sick in order to take a day off to rest, follow nursing procedures, etc.). Thus some respondents suspected that the survey was intended to trick them into admitting errors, and they refused to complete it. The investigators also felt that social desirability might have biased the responses to reflect how participants thought they should behave, rather than how they actually behaved. However, it was also reported that the focus group discussions which were held after the NUCAT-2 survey confirmed the results.

# The Practice Culture Questionnaire

The Practice Culture Questionnaire (PCQ) is being developed by Leicester University's clinical governance research and development unit to 'reveal aspects of practice culture that may be linked to a resistance to engage with clinical governance activities' (Stevenson, 2000). The PCQ consists of 25 statements about practice relating to qualities exhibited by successful commercial organisations (e.g. shared objectives, and routine performance measurement). The developers claim that the questionnaire gives access to employees' tacit assumptions by assessing 12 primary care issues within the context of clinical governance.

Respondents to the PCQ are asked to rate their agreement with each statement on a 4-point scale, with an extra response option for 'unsure'. The completed questionnaires are analysed to produce a team average (median) culture score and its culture spread score (range of scores excluding the lowest and highest scores). The culture spread score should reveal the level of cohesion within the team's responses. The developers hope that the PCQ may help primary care groups to identify areas of practice resistant to clinical governance and assist in the selection of appropriate change strategies.

So far the PCQ has been used in two primary care groups in Nottingham (40 practice teams) and seven primary care groups in Avon (70 practice teams). Validation work on its ability to identify strong cohesive teams with positive attitudes or resistance to clinical governance is to be conducted with Leicestershire primary care groups. Work is also in progress to compare practice performance data with practice PCQ scores. Reliability is tested through splithalf reliability within the questionnaire itself as 12 items are repeated.*

The PCQ addresses practice culture only in so far as this is defined by the clinical governance strategy. Although clinical governance marks an important development in NHS policy and perhaps also in practice, and is therefore relevant to culture, it is only one new and developing perspective. The PCQ is more accurately a clinical governance questionnaire. It does not address a broad view of organisational culture, nor is it aimed at the level of basic assumptions that define culture. The PCQ is included in this section primarily because it is being developed in NHS organisations and it focuses on an intended cultural shift towards the adoption of clinical governance.

# Mackenzie's Culture Questionnaire

Mackenzie (1995) devised a questionnaire to survey the organisational culture in four strategic business units (directorates) of an NHS trust. A questionnaire was constructed that consisted of 76 statements covering the following 12 dimensions of culture:

1 employee commitment
2 attitudes to and beliefs about innovation
3 attitudes towards change
4 the style of conflict resolution
5 the management style
6 confidence in the leadership
7 openness and trust
8 teamwork and co-operation
9 action orientation
10 human resource orientation
11 consumer orientation
12 organisational direction.

---

* K Stevenson, personal communication.

Forced-choice items were used, with respondents being asked to tick every statement which they felt was broadly true of their organisation. The questionnaire was piloted on a small group of staff from one directorate. Other data collection methods that were utilised included in-depth group interviews, norms listing and metaphorical analogies. A purposive sample of 30 staff from each directorate was sought. Each directorate was asked to supply the following volunteers: one group of six managers; one group of six newcomers; three groups of six staff consisting of a mixture of senior secretaries, staff representatives, 'old-timers', and men and women from support services and direct patient care jobs. This would provide a total sample of 120 individuals from the trust. In the event, a total of 107 staff were surveyed. No validity or reliability figures for this instrument have been reported.

# The Core Employee Opinions Questionnaire

The Core Employee Opinions Questionnaire (CEOQ) was developed by the Gallup Organisation (Buckingham and Coffman, 2000). The 13 core statements of which the CEOQ is comprised evolved from a number of quantitative and qualitative studies on the nature of 'productive work groups' and 'productive individuals', undertaken by Gallup researchers. In developing the CEOQ, the Gallup researchers focused on 'the consistently important human resource issues on which managers can develop specific action plans'.

The questionnaire covers the following 13 areas:

1 overall satisfaction with the organisation
2 the degree of clarity of understanding of work expectations
3 access to materials and equipment needed to do work
4 opportunities to do what the person does best
5 recognition and praise for good performance over the previous week
6 quality of caring relationship with supervisor
7 encouragement with regard to self-development
8 perceptions of how much opinions count
9 relationship between mission of organisation and feelings that one's job is important
10 fellow employees' commitment to ensuring 'quality' work
11 having a 'best friend' in the organisation
12 feedback on personal progress over the previous 6 months
13 opportunities to 'learn and grow' over the last year.

Respondents are requested to complete each question using a 5-point scale (where 5 = 'strongly agree' with statement and 1 = 'strongly disagree'). The Gallup researchers conducted a meta-analysis of data accumulated across 28 studies in order to examine the following two hypotheses.

1 Employee perceptions of quality of management practices measured by the 13 core items are related to business unit outcomes.
2 The validity of employee perceptions of quality of management practices measured by the 13 core items can be generalised across the organisations studied.

Data were aggregated at the business unit level and correlated with the following four aggregate performance measures:

- customer satisfaction/loyalty
- profitability
- productivity
- turnover.

The meta-analysis included the following individual studies linking employee perceptions with performance outcomes:

- 18 studies explored the relationship between business unit employee perceptions and customer perceptions
- 14 studies examined the relationship between employee perceptions and profitability
- 15 studies included measures of productivity
- 15 studies examined the relationship between employee perceptions and turnover.

The studies that were meta-analysed involved 105 680 individual employee responses to surveys and 2528 business units, representing an average of 42 employees per business unit and 90 business units per company (Buckingham and Coffman, 2000).

**Table 2.2:** Related items that can be generalised across organisations (reproduced with permission from Buckingham and Coffman, 2000)

| Core item | Customer | Profitability | Productivity | Turnover |
|---|---|---|---|---|
| 1 Overall satisfaction | | × | × | × |
| 2 Know what is expected | × | × | × | × |
| 3 Materials/equipment | | | × | × |
| 4 Opportunity to do what I do best | × | × | | × |
| 5 Recognition and praise | × | × | × | |
| 6 Cares about me | × | × | × | × |
| 7 Encourages development | | × | × | |
| 8 Opinions count | | × | × | |
| 9 Mission and purpose | | | × | |
| 10 Committed to quality | | × | × | |
| 11 Best friend | × | | × | |
| 12 Talked about progress | × | | × | |
| 13 Opportunities to learn and grow | | × | | |

Table 2.2 provides a summary of the items that were found to have a positive relationship with the four performance domains, and which were thought to be generalisable across organisations.

# General themes and issues that cut across the eight instruments

## How can culture be measured?

Measuring, assessing or describing organisational culture is a project beset with difficulties. Does one adopt an objective or an interpretive approach to data collection? How many respondents will be needed to represent the organisation as a whole – and its constituent occupational groups? Should data be sought only from top management, or from a wider range of respondents? These are all questions that can only be answered by 'It depends...'. It depends on what is meant by 'culture' and 'measurement', the purpose of the research, who wants to know about the culture and what they are going to do with the information, what resources are available for the investigation, and so on. However, some general observations and guidelines can be formulated.

We note first that the logical-positivist, quasi-experimental designs proposed by Cook and Campbell (1979) are broadly rejected by organisational culture researchers in favour of more qualitative, interpretative methods (Ott, 1989). Secondly, the general rule for organisational research is *horses for courses*. A design that works well for one investigation may not be so effective for another. There is an unfortunate tendency among some consultants and researchers to assume that one instrument or method is applicable to any problem or organisation. There are practical and theoretical arguments against that assumption. As a basic example, some organisations (such as the NHS) are widely dispersed geographically. For these organisations, large-scale data collection methods that require face-to-face contact between researchers and respondents might not be practicable, and an appropriate postal survey instrument might be more effective. However, if members of the study population have recently been asked to complete other survey questionnaires, a low response rate might be obtained. Thus the choice of research methods should take into account the characteristics and circumstances of the specific organisation or group.

Careful consideration should be given to what type of data is really needed and how best to obtain it. For some questions, data might already be accessible in the form of routinely collected statistics (Singh, 1998). For other questions, a unique data collection instrument might have to be designed and tested.

Between these two extremes there usually lies a middle ground consisting of the methods that other investigators have used for similar projects. This appears to be the case for organisational culture. An eclectic approach is also possible, whereby individually validated scales from one or more than one instrument are combined to form a hybrid data collection tool. For example, Ingersoll *et al.* (2000) utilise only three of the scales from Pasmore's Sociotechnical Systems Assessment Survey (STSAS) (Pasmore, 1988).

But do the available instruments really measure what we are interested in? The culture assessment tools surveyed cover a wide range of methodological approaches, from loosely structured interviews through projective metaphors to sophisticated questionnaires, but do any of them actually measure culture? If organisational culture is defined as espoused beliefs and values, there is no shortage of tools available. However, espoused beliefs and values, especially those concerning employees' opinions about the organisation, tend to measure organisational climate rather than culture. If, on the other hand, organisational culture is defined as the basic underlying assumptions that inform organisational beliefs, values and behaviour, the list of appropriate instruments is drastically shortened. In fact, it is unlikely that any instrument alone could measure culture defined in this way, even if it purported to do so.

This means that any method of assessing organisational culture is going to require considerable skill by investigators in either designing instruments to elicit tacit assumptions, or interpreting patterns of responses in terms of their expression of those assumptions. Working with ambiguous data demands more than one data collection method, so that results can be cross-checked or 'triangulated'. For example, in his study of Jones & Jones, Ott (1989) utilised Harrison's culture questionnaire (Harrison, 1975) and Alexander's organisational norms opinionnaire and ethnographic techniques (Alexander, 1978). The order in which multiple methods are administered can be important. Ott avoided contaminating his ethnographic research by not unsealing the completed questionnaires until he had spent three months observing life in the firm.

If we consider the view universally held by Jones & Jones employees, that all their customers are *'assholes'*, some inherent limitations of closed-question survey instruments become clear. None of the instruments that we have identified asks respondents whether they perceive their clients in quite those terms, nor could any instrument elicit an explanation of what the precise term meant in the context of the firm's culture. This example shows how easily conversations with employees can reveal a very different view of an organisation to that obtained by questionnaires.

This suggests that culture rating scales should be regarded as relatively insensitive, only capable of hinting at the underlying assumptions that give rise to the more easily accessible cultural artefacts, beliefs and values. The informing assumptions might only emerge through dialogue about participants' experiences, thoughts, attitudes and beliefs about the organisation.

Adopting an archaeological analogy, cultural artefacts may be found on the surface of the ground, like old coins or pottery shards. These fragments hint at what could lie below. Aerial photography might reveal the shape of ramparts, or the outline of a building, analogous to the cultural values that are held and sometimes espoused by organisational members. This outline might suggest the typical shape of an ancient settlement or Roman villa, but the underlying construction, of which these fragments and outlines of a culture are merely outward signs, has to be dug for carefully and without destruction. Only after the site has been thoroughly excavated can the buried walls or foundations upon which the superstructure once sat be revealed and understood.

The objection might be raised that an organisation's culture is a living system, not a relic of the past. In fact, a culture is both and neither of these. It is a living summary of an organisation's history, an accumulated residue of past behaviours, values and assumptions which have influenced its course in the past and which provide a pattern for the future. The principles of initially surveying the site/culture, forming hypotheses about the underlying assumptions, and then conducting a 'dig' to unearth those hidden secrets appear to be applicable. In practical terms, cultural assumptions might emerge gradually. Perhaps through the course of several encounters, the investigator hopes to inspire sufficient confidence for respondents to lower their guard and begin to divulge what they *really* think and feel about things. Goffman (1959) expresses this succinctly by making a distinction between a person's 'public face' and their 'private face'. Our public face refers to what we show and say to strangers such as researchers and consultants. Our private face refers to what we divulge to friends and confidants, and is nearer to our deeper thoughts, sentiments and beliefs. As most NHS staff of all occupations learn to be adept at dealing with the public, they might be expected to have readily available 'public faces' which they 'switch' on and off instinctively when approached by an outsider, or when completing a questionnaire. Getting behind the mask of the public face can be one of the most difficult challenges of culture research. Even then, respondents cannot be expected to articulate the unspoken assumptions that inform their values and guide their behaviour. As the quotation from Bateson (1941) in Part 1 suggested, a culture does not usually yield up its meanings or secrets easily.

# Other methods and approaches to organisational culture assessment

The methods described above are a collection of potentially useful sources to guide the assessment of health service organisational cultures. However, they are not intended to limit the instrument designer's choice, and reference to the alternative methods is strongly recommended. Although most of them have no track record of use in healthcare organisations, some appear to have good face value. For example, the use of projective metaphor, drawings and imagery by Lisney and Allen (1993) and Nossiter and Biberman (1990) appears to offer direct access to respondents' unconscious representations of their experience of their organisation. Discussion of this imagery might lead to an unearthing of unspoken assumptions more quickly than would be achieved by negotiating the complex maze of argot and slang that constitutes the linguistic dimension of organisations — and research.

Another example is Corzine's review of Machiavellianism and management (Corzine, 1997), which serves to highlight the organisational underworld of hidden motives and agendas, duplicity and manipulation, back-stabbing and secret struggles, suspicion, paranoia and even sadism — all of which are part and parcel of everyday life in the organisational jungle. These behaviours surely point to some of the less noble cultural values and assumptions in organisations, even in health services. Is ruthless ambition scarcer in public service organisations than in any other sector? Probably not — perhaps the Machiavellis of the NHS have to be even more cunning, even more Machiavellian, in order to conceal their dark thoughts and deeds behind an even more convincing public face. The availability of widely administered instruments to assess Machiavellianism thus offers a tempting opportunity to augment any culture rating scale.

# Summary of main points to be addressed when developing an organisational culture assessment tool

From the foregoing account we are now in a position to profile a desirable approach to health organisation culture assessment.

1 *Levels of culture.* The approach would be able to discriminate between different levels of culture — artefacts, values and assumptions. It would be capable of moving between these levels as an historian moves between sources to corroborate one with another. The flexible use of inductive and hypothetico-deductive methods would be needed. For example, identification of an espoused value such as 'We believe in patient-centred care' would trigger a search for artefacts, such as attitudes and practices in dealing with patients, and also a search for tacit assumptions, such as a shared expectation that other departments in the same organisation hold a similar value and act accordingly. If it is found that the value holder does not assume that others hold the same value, then that value cannot be regarded as being representative of the unit or organisation. If artefacts do not appear to support

the patient-centred care value, then this discrepancy is a further clue to the presence of an incongruent unspoken assumption.

2 *Triangulation.* The principle of multi-method assessment is implied in the previous point about corroborating one data source with another. For instance, artefacts could be recorded using observational techniques, values could be collected by questionnaire, and assumptions could be identified through interviews. The choice of method should be determined by the type of data needed within the overall context of the research.

3 *Sampling.* Sample pattern and size need to be considered. How many respondents are needed and from what range of occupational and other groups? If the aim is to map the cultural landscape of the system, a large study population would be needed in order to be representative of the whole organisation. Purposive sampling may be used to draw participants from specific locations. One method could be to recruit a proportion of participants from the same occupational groups at each location. For example, if at location A the ratio of managers to doctors is $1:4$ and the ratio of doctors to nurses is $1:3$, then the sample from that location could consist of 3 managers, 12 doctors and 36 nurses (plus other occupational groups).

The main method or instrument must therefore be capable of collecting data efficiently from such a sample. This suggests a questionnaire instrument, but it is likely that a commercial package such as the Organisational Culture Inventory (OCI) would be too expensive to use exclusively for that purpose. Possibly a subsample could be surveyed with this instrument. In addition to the question of how to obtain data, other questions need to be considered. Can existing data be accessed? How should one approach employees? Why should they help with the research? How might their co-operation be enhanced? How researched is the target population? Will their response rates be affected by research fatigue? Some investigators alienate their respondents, thereby reducing the opportunities for further research. It pays to find out who else has researched recently in which locations. Data can sometimes be exchanged between projects, although the original ethics permissions and consents must be respected.

Many health service employees already feel over-stretched with work demands, organisational changes and staff shortages. They will probably have faced more than one organisational development programme in recent years. Therefore we should expect to encounter some cynicism about a perceived 'hidden agenda' to a project investigating the organisation's culture and performance. Thus empirical research would need sensitive handling in order to avoid a dismissive response from some occupational groups. One way of handling resistance would be to formulate in advance the ways in which each occupational group might benefit from participation. For some groups this might need to be explained squarely in terms of benefits to patients. Some employees will suspect that the real motive behind the research is to cut jobs. This in itself indicates an important underlying assumption that researchers and consultants are merely agents of management.

4 *Analysis by occupational group.* The importance of occupational subculture is supported by Litwinenko and Cooper's study (Litwinenko and Cooper, 1994). It is important to choose data collection methods that allow both occupational-group and whole-group analysis. The characteristics of occupational groups may need to be factored into the design of the investigation/data collection (e.g. different locations, occupations, shift patterns, etc.). In a geographically dispersed system, each location might have a distinctive climate and possibly a distinctive culture. The research should therefore look for commonalities and differences between locations, especially in terms of underlying cultural assumptions. Different patterns of assumptions might be related to the local configuration of occupational groups.

5 *Collective unit of analysis.* Because culture is a shared phenomenon, the unit of analysis should be collective rather than individual. Individual data can be collected, but the method of aggregation should be validated (Shortell *et al.*, 1994).

6 *Culture and performance.* Finally, organisational culture assessment can allow meaningful comparison with organisational performance. However, an important issue concerns cultural assumptions about what performance means in the health system in question. Does it mean accurate identification of health improvement needs, a good match between epidemiological data/demographics and service provision, economic efficiency, better health outcomes, patient satisfaction, or a good quality of working life? A distinction needs to be made between responses that are contaminated by policy demands (e.g. performance indicators) and the deeper concerns and assumptions that participants might hold about the basic purpose and philosophy of the system. If these underlying cultural assumptions differ between occupational groups, they might be an important source of conflict between commitment to official strategic concerns and actual working practices.

# PART 3

# Culture and performance

## Introduction

Corporate or organisational culture has been used to explain the exceptional economic success of certain countries, including Japan and South Korea, compared with others, including America and the UK (Hofstede, 1980; Ouchi, 1981; Denison, 1984; Hofstede and Bond, 1988). These cultural comparisons are not novel, as relationships between attitudes to work and leisure and economic structures and performance have long been considered to be bound up with national or tribal cultures. The organisational culture perspective extends that anthropological perspective to explain differences in performance between different organisations within the same national culture (Peters and Waterman, 1982; Schein, 1985). Peters and Waterman (1982) claim to have determined the corporate cultural characteristics that lead to 'excellence'. Ouchi and Wilkins (1985) explain a relationship between corporate culture and productivity, while Deal and Kennedy (1982) claim to have found a link between 'strong' cultures and high levels of corporate performance.

Yet is there any hard evidence to support these claims for a link between organisational culture and performance? In the final part of this book, the relationship between organisational culture and performance is examined in the light of empirical research. We begin by looking briefly at the results of studies of organisational culture and performance in sectors other than healthcare. Next the results of culture and performance studies in healthcare organisations are examined in more detail. Some critical issues pertaining to the possible nature of the relationship between organisational culture and performance are then discussed. Finally, a summary of the main points to address when assessing links between health systems culture and performance is presented. The overall aim is to discover not only whether there is a demonstrable link between organisational culture and performance, and the nature of such a link if one exists, but also which *aspects* of culture appear to be most salient to investigating a link.

# Methodology

We employed a comprehensive electronic search to uncover all of the major pieces of empirical research examining a culture–performance link in health-care organisations. We began by searching the following databases for articles on organisational culture: Medline, Cinahl, King's Fund, Helmis and Dhdata. These databases combine coverage of all of the major English-language man-agement journals with an emphasis on health services research. The initial key search term was simply 'culture', but this was later refined to 'organisational culture' (and variants) in order to remove a large number of false hits referring to microbiological cultures. A cross-check on a 20% sample of records which had been retrieved confirmed that all of the relevant studies which had been located using the inclusive term were also located using the more restrictive term.

# Results

Of a total of 68 articles that appeared to report empirical studies of organisa-tional culture and performance, 18 relevant studies were identified (*see* Table 3.1).* Of these, nine have been conducted in non-healthcare organisations, and nine in healthcare organisations (one of them in the UK). The studies differ in terms of organisations, participants, levels of culture and performance and methodologies used. This variety of approaches is not surprising, as the per-formance measures generally relate to goals that are relevant to the specific organisation examined (Lim, 1995). Thus, the indicators used include indices of service quality in hospitals (Argote, 1989), cost per ton of newsprint (Frame *et al.*, 1989), returns on investment, equity and sales (Denison, 1984), hospital employee loyalty and commitment (Gerowitz *et al.*, 1996), the amount of money raised for a fundraising campaign (Rousseau, 1990), and risk-adjusted clinical outcomes for coronary artery bypass graft (CABG) patients (Shortell *et al.*, 2000). Variations in studies were also found with regard to the levels and aspects of culture measured. Thus cultural factors included mission state-ments (Frame *et al.*, 1989) and other artefacts (Quick, 1992), behaviour patterns (Nystrom, 1993; Rizzo *et al.*, 1994) and norms (Argote, 1989; Rousseau, 1990; Cameron and Freeman, 1991; Nystrom, 1993; Zimmerman *et al.*, 1994; Banerjee,

---

*We have not included in this section the research undertaken by the Gallup Organisation, which looked at the association between core employees' opinions and business outcomes (Buckingham and Coffman, 2000). This is because we only had access to the findings of a meta-analysis of 28 studies, rather than reports on individual studies. This meant that we could not distinguish between healthcare and non-healthcare studies which comprised the meta-analysis. The findings of the meta-analysis are presented in Part 2, Table 2.2 (*see* p. 93).

1995; Gerowitz *et al.*, 1996; Gerowitz, 1998), awards, ceremonies and rituals (Zimmerman *et al.*, 1993), and employee attitudes, beliefs and values (Frame *et al.*, 1989; Quick, 1992; Fairfield-Sonn, 1993; Zimmerman *et al.*, 1993; Lewis, 1994; Jackson, 1997; Shortell *et al.*, 2000). Global measures, including strength, fitness and adaptability of culture (Kotter and Heskett, 1992), were also assessed. Variations were also found with regard to the use of longitudinal (e.g. Denison, 1984) and cross-sectional (e.g. Rousseau, 1990) data on performance, and between ideographic (e.g. Frame *et al.*, 1989; Jackson, 1997) and nomothetic (e.g. Argote, 1989) study designs (Lim, 1995).* Nine studies found plausible evidence to support a link between organisational culture and performance (Denison, 1984; Argote, 1989; Frame *et al.*, 1989; Cameron and Freeman, 1991; Kotter and Heskett, 1992; Banerjee, 1995; Gerowitz *et al.*, 1996; Jackson, 1997; Gerowitz, 1998). Nine studies did not find plausible evidence for a link between organisational culture and performance (Rousseau, 1990; Quick, 1992; Fairfield-Sonn, 1993; Nystrom, 1993; Zimmerman *et al.*, 1993; Lewis, 1994; Rizzo *et al.*, 1994; Zimmerman *et al.*, 1994; Shortell *et al.*, 2000).

# Non-healthcare studies

Nine case studies were found that related to organisational culture and performance in non-healthcare organisations. They included four ideographic studies (Frame *et al.*, 1989; Quick, 1992; Fairfield-Sonn, 1993; Lewis, 1994) and five nomothetic studies (Denison, 1984; Rousseau, 1990; Cameron and Freeman, 1991; Kotter and Heskett, 1992; Banerjee, 1995). All of them assessed the impact of organisational culture on performance, three in the context of major organisational change programmes (Frame *et al.*, 1989; Fairfield-Sonn, 1993; Lewis, 1994). Of the nine studies, two examined culture level 1 (artefacts) (Frame *et al.*, 1989; Quick, 1992), four examined level 1a (behaviour patterns) (Denison, 1984; Frame *et al.*, 1989; Rousseau, 1990; Lewis, 1994), and all nine examined level 2 (attitudes, beliefs and values). None of the studies examined level 3 (underlying assumptions). Various specific culture factors and performance outcomes were examined using different instruments.

---

* The ideographic approach to social science research is based on the view that one can only understand the social world by gaining first-hand knowledge of the subject under investigation. Emphasis is placed on the analysis of subjective accounts generated by getting inside the organisation. The nomothetic approach to research emphasises systematic protocol and technique. It is epitomised by the methods of the natural sciences, which focus on testing hypotheses in accordance with the canons of scientific rigour (Burrell G and Morgan G (1979) *Sociological Paradigms and Organisational Analysis*. Gower, Aldershot).

**Table 3.1:**  Studies of the relationship between organisational culture and performance

| Study | Participants | Context | Culture levels | Culture instruments | Performance indicators | Summary of findings |
|---|---|---|---|---|---|---|
| **Non-healthcare studies** | | | | | | |
| Fairfield-Sonn (1993) USA Ideographic | Employees of 'Weston' Town Council | A two-and-a-half-year change programme | Level 2: attitudes, beliefs and values | Questionnaire survey instrument, including essay (post-test) | Combined with culture questionnaire/essay | No objective data Survey results do not support a link between culture change and performance |
| Frame *et al.* (1989) USA Ideographic | Managers of the *Chicago Tribune* printing plant | The paper had sacked 1000 striking workers and recruited a new and inexperienced workforce | Level 1: mission statements Level 1a: behaviour patterns Level 2: attitudes, beliefs and values | Employee survey (pre-test) | Cost per ton of newsprint Productivity Reliability Quality Bonuses | The drastic performance improvements achieved tend to support a culture–performance link |
| Lewis (1994) Australia Ideographic | Staff of 'ATISIA' (Australian college) | Transformation of ATISIA college into a university | Level 1a: behaviour patterns Level 2: attitudes, beliefs and values | Ethnographic interviews, focus groups, observation | Income Student statistics Organisational goals | No evidence for a link between values and performance was found: values were eroded, yet performance improved |
| Quick (1992) USA Ideographic | Southwest Airlines | Influence of the founder | Level 1: artefacts created by the leader Level 2: values | Unclear | Services opened Quality awards Passenger figures Productivity Union/employee relations | Anecdotal evidence presented for a link between the founder of the culture and performance |

| | | | | | | |
|---|---|---|---|---|---|---|
| Banerjee (1995)<br>USA<br>Nomothetic | 188 administrative-level personnel employed by a state welfare department | Examines multivariate relationships between competing values effectiveness, job satisfaction, client centredness and service outcome | Level 2: attitudes, beliefs and values | Competing values effectiveness was measured by means of the competing values framework (Quinn, 1988). Job satisfaction was measured by means of a job satisfaction index (Poertner *et al.* (unpublished). Client centredness was measured by a client centredness index | Service outcomes were measured using a 5-item scale: (1) service enables clients to return to normal living, (2) service delivery is reliable, (3) services are delivered courteously, (4) services are delivered indiscriminately, (5) services are delivered with an eye to client satisfaction | Competing values effectiveness and client centredness together were found to predict service outcomes with standardised regression beta weights of 0.43 and 0.25, respectively. Job satisfaction showed a strong correlation with competing values effectiveness, but only a weak independent relationship with service outcomes |
| Cameron and Freeman (1991)<br>USA<br>Nomothetic | 3406 individuals at 334 colleges and universities in the USA | Examines the relationship between the congruence, strength and type of organisational cultures and organisational effectiveness | Level 2: attitudes, beliefs and values | Competing values framework | Organisational effectiveness (Cameron, 1978, 1981, 1986) Organisational structure (Mintzberg, 1979; Weik, 1976) Student career development Organisational strategic orientations (Miles and Cameron, 1982; Miles and Snow, 1978) Decision-making processes (Nutt, 1976) Organisational saga and mission (Clarke, 1970) and environmental conditions (Wilkins and Ouchi, 1983) | A link between type of culture and effectiveness is supported (links between strength of culture and congruence of culture are not supported) |

*(continued)*

**Table 3.1:** *(continued)*

| Study | Participants | Context | Culture levels | Culture instruments | Performance indicators | Summary of findings |
|---|---|---|---|---|---|---|
| Denison (1984) USA Nomothetic | Respondents ($n = 43\,747$) from 6671 workgroups in 34 companies | Study comparing archive culture data with standard and poor COMPUSTAT data | Levels 1a and 2: perceptions of work design, leadership, group functioning and satisfaction | 125-item 'Survey of Organisations' | Return on investment, equity and sales | The results presented tend to support a link between climate/culture and performance. Only a part of the results is reported |
| Kotter and Heskett (1992) Nomothetic | 207 American companies and 75 industry financial analysts | Longitudinal study of relationships between culture and performance | Level 2: strength of corporate culture; cultural beliefs, including fitness | Strength of culture survey Culture content survey Interviews on culture history and change | Average yearly increases in net income, return on investment, and increase in stock price | The findings do not support a link between strong culture and performance |
| Rousseau (1990) USA Nomothetic | Permanent staff ($n = 263$) in 32 units of a voluntary service organisation | Executive development programme | Levels 1a and 2: behavioural norms and normative beliefs | Organizational Culture Inventory (Cooke and Lafferty, 1987) | Archive data on community fundraising success | The findings do not generally support a link between culture and performance |
| **Healthcare studies** Jackson (1997) UK Ideographic | Staff of hospital outpatient department, and 35 'Did not attend' (DNA) patients | Study of the effect of hospital outpatient department culture on DNA rates | Level 1a: behaviour patterns Level 2: attitudes, values and beliefs | Non-participant observation and telephone survey | Number of patients who did not attend appointments | A link between culture and performance (DNAs) is supported |
| Argote (1989) USA Nomothetic | Physicians ($n = 463$) and nurses ($n = 278$) working in emergency units in 30 hospitals | Comparative study of the relationship between norms and work-unit effectiveness | Level 1a: behavioural norms | Normative complementarity (agreement between groups) Normative consensus (agreement within groups) | Work-unit effectiveness, including promptness of care, quality of nursing care and quality of medical care | The results tend to support a link between culture and performance |

| Study | Sample | Purpose | Level | Instruments | Performance measures | Findings |
|---|---|---|---|---|---|---|
| Gerowitz et al. (1996) USA, UK and Canada Nomothetic | Top management teams of 265 hospitals (120 in the USA, 100 in UK, and 45 in Ontario, Canada) | Comparative study of top management culture and hospital performance | Level 2: values | Competing values framework (Cameron and Freeman, 1991) | Employee loyalty and commitment, external stakeholder satisfaction, internal consistency, external resource acquisition and overall adaptability | As hypothesised, the dominant culture of the hospital management team was positively and significantly related to organisational performance. A link between culture and performance is supported |
| Gerowitz (1998) USA Nomothetic | Top management teams of 120 hospitals in the USA ($n = 271$) | Study to assess the impact of TQM/CQI interventions on the culture and performance of top management teams | Level 2: values | Competing values framework (Cameron and Freeman, 1991) | Adaptability and global performance were measured subjectively by managers | A link between culture and performance is partially supported – culture focus and culture orientation both accounted for significant variations in performance differences |
| Nystrom (1993) USA Nomothetic | 41 senior managers and 36 executive secretaries in 13 healthcare organisations | Study of impact of culture on organisational commitment, job satisfaction and performance, and relationship between strategy and culture | Level 1a: norms Level 2: satisfaction, commitment and values | Kilmann-Saxton Culture-Gap Survey (Kilmann and Saxton, 1983) Managerial values questionnaire (England and Keaveny, 1969) Organisational commitment questionnaire (Moday et al., 1979) Job Diagnostic Survey (Hackman and Oldham, 1975) | Managers' judgements comparing the overall performance of their organisation with that of other organisations producing similar products or services | A link between culture and performance is claimed, but there are methodological problems |

(continued)

**Table 3.1:** (*continued*)

| Study | Participants | Context | Culture levels | Culture instruments | Performance indicators | Summary of findings |
|---|---|---|---|---|---|---|
| Rizzo *et al.* (1994) USA Nomothetic | 235 nursing department staff from 13 units | Analysis of nursing unit culture and work characteristics to inform change in care delivery model | Level 1a: behaviour patterns | Nursing Unit Cultural Assessment Tool (NUCAT-2) (Coeling and Simms, 1993) | Unit skill mix Cost measures Worked hours per patient day Quality assurance monitors Documentation of care planning and discharge planning Patient satisfaction | Only one unit had reached its 1-year evaluation mark. It is unclear whether a link between culture and performance is supported or not |
| Shortell *et al.* (2000) USA Nomothetic | 3045 CABG patients from 16 hospitals | To assess the impact of TQM and organisational culture on organisational performance | Level 2: attitudes, beliefs and values | 20-item version of the competing values framework (Cameron and Freeman, 1991) | Risk-adjusted clinical outcomes, functional health status, patient satisfaction and cost measures | A link between culture and performance is not generally supported |
| Zimmerman *et al.* (1993) USA Ideographic and nomothetic | 3672 ICU admissions, 316 nurses and 202 physicians | To examine organisational practices associated with higher and lower ICU performance | Level 1: awards and ceremonies Level 1a: rituals, learning and teaching Level 2: attitudes, beliefs and values | Interviews and direct observations Organisational Culture Inventory (Cooke and Lafferty, 1987; Cooke and Rousseau, 1988) | Effectiveness was measured by the ratio of actual/predicted hospital deaths Efficiency was measured by the ratio of actual/predicted length of ICU stay | Structural and organisational questionnaires, self-evaluation by staff members, and the research team's implicit judgements following detailed on-site analysis failed to distinguish between higher and lower performing units. A link between culture and performance is not supported |

| Zimmerman et al. (1994) USA Ideographic and nomothetic | 888 ICU admissions, 70 nurses and 42 physicians | To examine structural and organisational characteristics, including culture, at two ICUs with marked differences in risk-adjusted survival | Level 1a: behavioural norms | Creativity, task preferences, communication style and mutual support were measured by an (unnamed) organisational and managerial process questionnaire | Risk-adjusted mortality ratio Mean actual to mean predicted ICU length-of-stay ratio Mean actual to mean predicted ICU resource utilisation ratio Self-evaluated technical quality of care On-site investigator ranking | Structural and organisational questionnaires, self-evaluation by staff members, and the research team's implicit judgements following detailed on-site analysis failed to distinguish between higher and lower performing units. A link between culture and performance is not supported |

# Ideographic non-healthcare studies

Frame *et al.* (1989) describe an organisational transformation intervention based on mission statements, behaviour patterns and attitudes, beliefs and values at a *Chicago Tribune* printing plant. Drastic improvements in productivity, quality and bonuses were all reported. However, the context of these performance improvements was unusual in that the plant had recently sacked 1000 striking workers and recruited a new and inexperienced workforce. Although the workplace culture therefore undoubtedly changed, and the performance improvements were doubtless linked to these changes, it is hard to attribute the performance improvements to formal cultural interventions by the consultants and management involved. No data are provided to show the extent to which the new cultural values were accepted or internalised by the workforce. Thus it seems likely that both culture change and performance improvements arose from the crisis triggered by the strike.* Frame *et al.* (1989) suggest that crisis and/or radical change may be necessary precursors to revolutions in organisational culture and performance. Whether the NHS is currently experiencing a comparable crisis is debatable and depends on one's point of view. Clearly the provocation of such a crisis is unthinkable. Thus although the *Chicago Tribune* study shows some kind of link between culture and performance, it offers little to inform a study of culture and performance in the public sector.

Quick (1992) studied the founder's role in disseminating the core values of humour and altruism at Southwest Airlines. Quick explains Southwest's success solely in terms of Herb Kelleher's influence. Figures are presented testifying to the commercial success of the airline, but no empirical connection between Herb Kelleher and his company's growth and quality achievements is demonstrated. The role of the founder in the early development of organisational cultures and in organisational performance are both established hypotheses (Pettigrew, 1979; Schein, 1985), but the connection between the two hypotheses is unclear. Quick merely trades on an assumed causality between them. No data are presented to show that Kelleher's values are shared by other organisational members.

Fairfield-Sonn (1993) examined the impact of a two-and-a-half-year organisational and culture change effort within a town council. The survey results suggested that the change effort had failed. However, as the culture change was not effectively disseminated, the study tells us little about the relationship between culture and performance. After two years of concentrated effort, only the senior management team had 'bought into' the new organisational values. Fairfield-Sonn draws five pithy lessons out of the exercise, which

---

*It is of course possible to provoke a walkout and use this as a pretext to sack strikers on the grounds of frustration of contract, and then to recruit a new workforce that is unaccustomed to the old 'restrictive practices'. This is one way of changing an organisation's culture.

although not new are worth repeating in the context of health systems culture and performance.

1  It is easier to develop a corporate culture ideal than to implement it. Stubborn resistance should be anticipated, particularly when the vision is provided by an outsider who tries to infuse it into an organisation.
2  When creating a new vision of the culture of an organisation, the values must be stated with respect to the existing culture, and combine end goals with means goals.
3  In conveying the new vision, leaders must either create conditions for change or take advantage of external threats to get their message across. A vision by itself will be insufficient to convince most employees of the need for change.
4  Cultural change efforts must be pursued with the intention of promoting simultaneous strategic and operational change (it is no good setting the signals to green if the track is not clear).
5  It is vital for change agents to continuously identify and refine their understanding of the forces that are promoting and inhibiting change.

(Adapted from Fairfield-Sonn, 1993, p. 53)

Lewis (1994) presents an informative account of a longitudinal case study of an institution undergoing transformation from an Australian college of education to a university. Like the *Chicago Tribune* printing plant (Frame *et al.*, 1989), ATISIA college underwent radical or 'transformative' change, defined by De Bivort (1985) as 'breaking through existing belief structures'. Lewis collected data on ATISIA's culture and performance, triangulating qualitative and quantitative methods, over a period of four years. Objective output as well as observational data were used as performance indicators, and were compared with information collected from interviews. Lewis found that staff work-related values in ATISIA contradicted staff behaviour and organisational performance. Although many staff professed to have lost their old values of teaching, industrial experience and professional bodies, ATISIA achieved university status, attracted better-quality students, accepted PhD students and received more government grants and external money. While many staff also professed to have lost the values of loyalty to ATISIA (trust, honesty and cohesion), many others showed evidence of negative work-related values:

> The study of ATISIA demonstrated that, in implementing change to achieve organisational effectiveness, it is necessary only to change patterned group behaviour, because in the *short term* at least, only behaviour can directly affect performance, and while behaviour may be one embodiment of culture, culture is certainly not the only determinant of behaviour.

(Lewis, 1994, p. 51, our italics)

Lewis's study suggests that staff can be persuaded and coerced to produce better organisational performance despite their values, at least in the short term. How long this dissonant situation could be sustained is another question. The study also suggests that the link between culture and performance is bidirectional:

> Instead of assuming that values cause the development of a certain behaviour, there is the possibility that behaviour causes the development of certain values.
>
> (Lewis, 1994, p.51)

Lewis (1994) examines the link between espoused values, behaviour patterns and effectiveness, and finds a complex and paradoxical relationship. Schein (1985) emphasises the value of using such discrepancies between espoused values and actual practices in seeking to unearth the underlying cultural assumptions which he regards as the *essence* of an organisation's culture. That exploration would almost certainly have helped the observer to make clearer sense of the dissonance between the old-established culture, the new up-and-coming culture, and the doubtless fought-over criteria of effectiveness that were chosen to signal success or failure in Lewis's study.

One commentator concludes that Lewis's ATISIA study (Lewis, 1994) suggests a negative or at best no relationship between culture and performance (Lim, 1995). Although it may be true that no simple causal relationship holds between culture and performance, surely the real challenge is to understand the complexity of a link that logically must exist. If organisational culture includes artefacts and behaviour (Schein, 1985; Ott, 1989) – that is, behaviour which is *performed* – then a proper definition of *culture* must include at least some elements of *performance*. Performance criteria and data are culturally defined. We can only keep the categories of culture and performance analytically distinct and comparable by placing them in different sets. This artificial arrangement allows us to ask the question 'Is there a relationship between organisational culture on the one hand and organisational performance on the other?'. The answer, as Wittgenstein observed, is contained in the question. If culture and performance are both *organisational*, then the question contains its own answer – culture and performance are two variables, dimensions or expressions of organisation. They must therefore exist in (an organisational) relationship. Whether culture and performance are subcategories of organisation, or whether the three terms are virtually interchangeable, as we suspect, is only one *ontological* aspect of their relationship. From a culture perspective we are more interested in the meaning with which these terms are invested, and we can only begin to understand the meaning of terms in relation to one another (Deleuze, 1990). Therefore on a *phenomenological–epistemological level*, too, the terms are firmly yet variably linked. On a *practical* level the link between culture and performance is equally strong because their association in organisational discourse alone affirms their perceptual and actual linkage. By saying that they are related and acting in accordance with the assertion, we make it so.

The real question that Lewis's study prompts us to ask then is not 'Is there a link?' but rather 'What are the operative links between organisational culture and performance?'. Because we have recognised throughout this account that a plurality of perspectives on organisational culture (and performance) exists, the question is immediately revised to 'Which links between organisational culture and performance do we perceive, mean, act on, etc.?'.

On balance, we conclude that only one (Frame *et al.*, 1989) of the four non-healthcare ideographic studies might demonstrate a link between organisational culture and performance. Unfortunately, due to the extreme change in the workforce, we are no clearer about the nature of that link.

# Nomothetic non-healthcare studies

Banerjee (1995) assessed the multivariate relationships between competing values effectiveness, job satisfaction, client centredness and service outcomes. Competing values effectiveness and client centredness together were found to predict service outcomes, supporting a link between the welfare department's culture and its performance. However, the claim that this approach to assessing effectiveness of outcomes 'brings clients centre-stage to our service delivery system' (Banerjee, 1995, p. 43) appears hollow in view of its exclusive reliance on service providers', not clients', assessment of service outcomes. To bring the clients 'centre-stage' while at the same time keeping them silent in the wings is an impressive theatrical feat. Once again Schein's methodology (Schein, 1985) of exploring the discrepancies (cracks in the façade?) between espoused values and actual practices appears apposite. Perhaps the contradiction about the central role of the client hints at another, role-focused side of the welfare department's culture.

Cameron and Freeman (1991) investigated the relationship between congruence, strength and type of organisational cultures and their effectiveness using the competing values framework (Quinn and Rohrbaugh, 1981). A comparison of the cultures of 334 higher education institutions found no significant differences between organisations with strong cultures compared with those with weak cultures. However, the study did find that the type of culture possessed by the organisation (clan, adhocracy, hierarchy or market) has an important relationship with effectiveness.

In one of the earliest quantitative studies of organisational culture and performance, Denison (1984) used archived questionnaire data to compare the culture and performance of 34 American firms over a five-year period. Responses to two indices relating to perceptions of work organisation and participation in decision making were correlated with data subsequently collected annually on return on investment and return on sales. A comparison was made between firms that were in the top half of the work organisation and participation indices and those that were in the lower half. Companies that were perceived as having a well-organised work environment showed consistently higher levels of performance in terms of both return on investment and return on sales than less well-organised firms. Decision-making styles were less clearly related to effectiveness, with similar returns on investment and sales over the first three study years, followed by a sudden marked improvement by the more participative firms in the fourth and fifth study years. A comparison between the study firms and the rest of their industry showed a similar pattern of results.

Denison's claim that organisation of work and decision-making practices impact on performance appears to be supported by these findings, but there is some cause for scepticism. In Part 2 we argued for the triangulation of results of more than one data collection method in order to improve the reliability of findings. We also noted that questionnaires might not be the most effective means of collecting data about the deeper levels of organisational culture. As Denison uses only two out of 22 scales on one instrument, his approach to measuring organisational culture is not very rigorous. Moreover, as Lim (1995) comments, employee perceptions of work organisation and participation are arguably measures of organisational *climate* rather than of culture. Thus while this study shows some correlation between perceptions of specific organisational factors and performance, it still falls short.

Kotter and Heskett (1992) studied the link between culture and performance in 207 firms over a five-year period. Their research was iterative, with the investigators building on earlier stages of the research, testing successively theoretical links between 'strong' cultures, strategically appropriate cultures and adaptive cultures. Only a modest correlation was found between strength of corporate culture and long-term performance. 'The statement "strong cultures create excellent performance" appears to be just plain wrong', according to Kotter and Heskett (1992, p. 21). The second phase of the research showed that firms with cultures that were well matched with their market context performed better than did those that also had strong cultures but were less well matched to their environment. Finally, in a follow-up study the authors found that firms which showed consistently good performance over time tended to possess core values that emphasised the importance of an adaptive culture.

Rousseau (1990) used the Organizational Culture Inventory (Cooke and Lafferty, 1987) to study the relationship between culture and performance in 32 units of a voluntary service organisation. The sole performance indicator was the amount of money raised by a recent fundraising campaign. No significant positive correlations were found between normative beliefs and outcomes, although a significant negative correlation was found between funds raised and people-security-oriented norms (approval, conventional and dependent). The failure to find a relationship could also have been due to the use of cross-sectional rather than longitudinal data (Lim, 1995).

Thus four studies (Denison, 1984; Cameron and Freeman, 1991; Kotter and Heskett, 1992; Banerjee, 1995) out of the five nomothetic non-healthcare studies yielded some evidence of a link between organisational culture and performance. Of the nine non-healthcare studies in total, therefore, five tend to support a link between culture and performance.

# Healthcare studies

## Ideographic healthcare studies

Jackson (1997) used non-participant overt observations of a hospital outpatient department to view the processes and attitudes of patients and staff during a typical outpatients session, and a telephone survey of patients/parents of patients who did not attend for their hospital paediatric outpatient appointment. The telephone survey also included a similar number of matched controls. The results of this study suggest that a relationship existed between the outpatient department's culture and patients' attendance, but that its precise nature was unclear. The key observations were that the overall culture was role oriented, not customer focused. The senior medical staff subculture emphasised personal prestige. Medical staff automatically requested further appointments for identified 'Did not attends' (DNAs), exacerbating DNA rates. Anecdotal evidence indicated that medical staff saw a more efficient NHS (including fewer DNAs) as a threat to their private practice uptake. There was also a lack of customer orientation, as telephones were not answered promptly and patients at the outpatients reception window were not attended to promptly. The consumer views collected showed that the majority of parents who attended were happy with the children's treatment and appointment system. However, one consumer complained that receptionists continued their social conversation instead of attending to patients at the reception window. In three DNA cases, 6-month follow-ups were arranged by junior doctors who may not have been competent to discharge these patients (Mason, 1992). Of 17 DNAs, three (18%) had transport problems, three (18%) tried to cancel but could not get through on the telephone, and 12 (70%) knew that they could not attend but made no effort to rearrange or cancel their appointment. Among these, the reasons for not contacting the hospital included the perception that changing appointments was discouraged by the hospital (one parent), and a failure to give their child an X-ray as promised at the previous appointment. Some appointments only involved weighing and measuring a child, which could have been done more conveniently at the GP surgery.

In Part 2 we argued that patients as well as practitioners should be included in a definition of health service organisational culture. Jackson's study (Jackson,

1997) supports this idea. The behaviour of patients is likely to be influenced by practitioners, and vice versa. If reception staff do not attend to patients promptly, this will affect patients' attitudes and may influence their attendance, which may in turn influence staff attitudes and behaviour towards patients, and so on. If an important part of health service culture concerns encounters between patients and staff, certain implications follow. One such implication is that it is impossible to reduce the culture's essence to the behaviour, values and assumptions of patients *or* practitioners – both must be brought into the equation. Another implication is that intervention on one side or the other (patients or practitioners) may be efficacious in changing the culture that is shared between them. We have perhaps seen this effect in recent years in patient–practitioner communication. Whether patients become more assertive or practitioners become better communicators, the effect is likely to be similar.

# Nomothetic healthcare studies

Argote (1989) examined the link between organisational culture and perform-ance by testing the relationship between organisational cultural norms and work-unit effectiveness in 44 hospital emergency units. Two dimensions of norm structures were analysed, namely *normative complementarity* (the amount of agreement *between groups* about norms governing their relationship; Georgo-poulos, 1965) and *normative consensus* (the amount of agreement that exists *within a group* about norms). Organisational effectiveness included three dimen-sions, namely promptness of care, quality of nursing care and quality of medi-cal care. As normative complementarity of care increased, promptness of care increased ($r(28) = 0.43; P < 0.05$), quality of nursing care increased ($r(28) = 0.39; P < 0.05$) and quality of medical care increased ($r(28) = 0.46; P < 0.01$). Similarly, as normative consensus increased, promptness of care increased ($r(28) = 0.39; P < 0.05$), quality of nursing care increased ($r(28) = 0.18$; non-significant) and quality of medical care increased ($r(28) = 0.34; P < 0.01$).

A regression analysis showed that normative complementarity and norma-tive consensus together explained a significant amount of variance in the effectiveness indicators. The coefficients of complementarity were positive and statistically significant in all three regressions, whereas the coefficient of con-sensus was not significant in any of the regressions. Additional equations were estimated, which included key control variables together with the norms variables as predictors of effectiveness. The coefficients of the complementarity variable in the three regressions were positive and statistically significant in all three regressions, whereas the coefficients of consensus were not significant in any of the regressions.

This study suggests that agreement about norms between groups is posit-ively and significantly associated with the effectiveness of emergency units. The relationship between normative agreement within units is weaker and less clear. Argote's 1989 results tend to agree with those of Krackhardt and Stern (1988), which found that organisations with strong between-group ties were more effective than organisations with strong within-group ties in crisis situations. As crises in emergency units are usual and therefore not 'crises' in the normal sense, Argote's findings suggest that a similar relationship between inter-group normative agreement and performance may also exist in non-critical situations.

One criticism of Argote's study (Argote, 1989) is that normative com-plementarity and consensus are both measured by nurses' opinions on how they perceive their job compared with how the hospital perceives their job. As has already been suggested, the independent variable represented by employees' perceptions and opinions is organisational climate rather than culture. The pre-cise relationship between climate and culture is unclear (Ott, 1989). Although it might appear reasonable to include climate under culture level 2 (attitudes, beliefs and values), one could equally well argue that employee normative per-ceptions and opinions of an organisation are level 1 artefacts. Climate might also conceivably yield clues to underlying assumptions. One way of approaching climate could be to regard it as a culture barometer which can give a quick predictive reading of organisational 'temperature' and 'pressure', but which is not as informative or reliable as a thorough professional 'forecast'.

Gerowitz et al. (1996) examined the role of top management team culture in a total of 265 hospitals located in Canada (45 hospitals), the UK (100 hospitals) and the USA (120 hospitals). The competing values framework (Cameron and Freeman, 1991) was used to identify clan, open, hierarchical and rational cul-tures. Three questions were addressed. First, do hospital management teams in the USA, Canada and the UK have different management cultures, given the differences in their political economies? Secondly, is management culture asso-ciated with differences in performance? Thirdly, is culture type a legitimate independent variable?

Their findings supported the premise that the political economy influences the distribution of culture types and the legitimacy of the cultural variable. The dominant cultures of the hospital management teams were positively and significantly related to organisational performance for clan, rational and open cultures. The Chi-square analysis of the distribution of culture types within each country was significant at the 0.05 level. Hospital management teams in the UK were more frequently clan and hierarchical cultures, those in the USA were more frequently rational and open cultures, and those in Canada were more frequently clan and rational cultures. Five performance measures were selected to assess the relationship between culture type and performance, namely employee loyalty, external stakeholder satisfaction, internal consistency, external resource acquisition and overall adaptability. The dominant culture of the hospital management team was positively and significantly related to organisational performance — *in the domain valued by the culture* — in the cases of clan, open and rational cultures. Hospitals with dominant clan cultures performed significantly above the mean on measures of employee loyalty and commitment in comparison with those with open, hierarchical and rational cultures ($x = 1.03$; sd $= 0.09$; $P = 0.03$).* Hospitals with dominant open cultures performed positively and significantly above the mean on the measure of external stakeholder satisfaction in comparison with clan, hierarchical and rational cultures ($x = 1.04$; sd $= 0.9$; $P = 0.02$).* The performance of hospitals with dominant hierarchical cultures was significantly different in the internal consistency domain from that of clan, rational and open cultures. However, the performance of hierarchical cultures on this measure was below the mean and therefore in the opposite direction of that postulated. Hierarchical cultures scored below the mean in areas related to cost containment and efficiency compared with open and rational cultures. Hospitals with dominant rational cultures performed above the mean in areas related to resource acquisition and competitiveness, and performed significantly better than those with dominant clan and hierarchical cultures.

The findings of Gerowitz *et al.* (1996) have implications for health policy. According to Lawrence and Dyer (1983), when firms are readaptive, achieving both efficiencies and innovation, there is no need for government intervention. However, if an industry becomes dominated by clan and/or hierarchical cultures, that industry may sub-optimise efficiency at the cost of lower innovation. Government policy makers may wish to intervene in such situations. An industry that sub-optimises innovation at the cost of low efficiency may also justify policy intervention. If, as the findings of Gerowitz *et al.* (1996) suggest, the NHS as a whole is characterised by a higher frequency of dominant clan and hierarchical cultures than of open or rational cultures, we would expect it to perform well in terms of employee loyalty and commitment, but not so well in terms of external stakeholder satisfaction, resource acquisition, competitiveness and internal consistency. Given these predictions, it would be fruitful to apply the competing values framework more widely to the NHS in order to examine whether the dominant culture types really are clan and hierarchical, and whether judgements about the performance of NHS organisations have the strengths and weaknesses that are predicted and valued by those culture types.

The competing values framework has a strong provenance in psychology and organisational research, and tries to match organisational culture with the performance criteria that are valued by that culture. It implies the question

---

* $x$ expresses the relationship between culture type and measures of performance, where $x = 1$ is the mean.

'Which organisational culture performance criteria are desired by society and policy makers?', rather than demanding an absolute choice by asking 'What is the best culture and performance for any society?'. By selecting a range of units of analysis, including different occupational groups, different types of NHS organisation and different parts of the UK, it might be possible to construct an accurate and useful picture of NHS culture and subcultures to compare with appropriate performance criteria.

In 1998, Gerowitz published another study, this time assessing the impact of TQM/CQI interventions on the culture and performance of the top management teams of 120 hospitals in the USA only (Gerowitz, 1998). The competing values framework was used to assess culture type, and the performance indicators measured were adaptability and global performance, as gauged subjectively by managers.

A Chi-square analysis was performed in order to determine any significant difference in the distribution of high- and low-performing organisations associated with TQM/CQI initiation. No significant differences were found. A second Chi-square analysis was performed to determine whether there was any significant difference in the distribution of high- and low-performing organisations associated with culture *focus* (internal clan and hierarchical cultures vs. external open and rational culture types). Significant differences in the distribution of high- and low-performing organisations associated with culture focus were found. Externally focused cultures were associated with high performance, whereas internally focused cultures were associated with low performance. A third Chi-square analysis was performed to determine whether there was any significant difference in the distribution of high- and low-performing organisations associated with culture *orientation* (mechanistic hierarchical and rational cultures vs. relational clan and open types). No significant association was found.

The results of a linear regression analysis indicated that TQM/CQI did not account for significant variance in performance. However, culture focus and culture orientation both accounted for significant variations in performance. High-performing organisations displayed open/rational cultures, whereas the low-performing organisations had clan/hierarchical cultures.

Along with its exclusive attention to USA hospitals, Gerowitz's 1998 study disconnects performance criteria from culture type, thereby losing some of the subtlety of their earlier comparative study (Gerowitz *et al.*, 1996). In the later study, performance was more narrowly defined in terms of the ability of organisations to anticipate and adapt to change, and the 'percent of ideal performance you feel that your firm is achieving in your industry' (Gerowitz, 1998, p. 4). This orientation towards the more competitive USA healthcare context makes translation of the findings to the NHS difficult, particularly as the frequencies of dominant organisational culture types in the UK (clan and hierarchical) were found to be different from those in the USA (more rational and open) in the 1996 study. However, in general terms, the 1998 findings support the view that as a hierarchical-clan culture the NHS is ill suited to operate in a competitive healthcare market.

Nystrom (1993) similarly focused on the higher echelons in a study of the impact of task norms (Kilmann and Saxton, 1983) and pragmatic values (England and Keaveny, 1969) on employee outcomes, including organisational commitment (Moday et al., 1979), job satisfaction (Hackman and Oldham, 1975) and performance. Performance was measured by asking managers to compare the overall performance of their organisation with that of other organisations which produced similar products or services (Pearce et al., 1987). The organisations were also classified according to strategic type (prospectors, analysers, defenders and reactors) (Miles and Snow, 1978). In total, 41 senior managers and 36 executive secretaries in 13 healthcare organisations in the USA were included in the study.

The results showed that culture did appear to affect employee outcomes and performance. Job satisfaction and organisational commitment both correlated significantly with task norms and pragmatic values. Job satisfaction correlated significantly with organisational commitment both for managers ($r = 0.77$; $P < 0.001$) and for executive secretaries ($r = 0.82$; $P < 0.001$). This was consistent with the results of Alpander's hospital study (Alpander, 1990), which showed significant correlations between satisfaction and commitment ($r = 0.53-0.69$; $P < 0.01$). The results also showed that organisational cultures differed for healthcare organisations that were pursuing alternative strategies. The distribution of task-norm scores for managers who saw their organisations pursuing a consistent strategy (prospectors, analysers or defenders) was compared with the distribution of task-norm scores for managers who saw their organisation operating with an inconsistent strategy (reactors). The organisations with an inconsistent strategy tended to exhibit weaker norms ($t = -2.11$, $P < 0.04$) and weaker values ($t = -1.97$, $P < 0.03$) than did the organisations that were pursuing any of the three consistent strategies.

According to Nystrom (1993) these results show that a stronger culture is more effective than a weaker one, but this conclusion does not follow directly from the data. The results show that when senior managers are strongly committed to their jobs and perceive the organisation's strategy to be coherent, they are more committed to the organisation and derive greater job satisfaction. However, the results tell us nothing about the relationship between an organisation's culture and its performance.

Rizzo et al. (1994) analysed the nursing-unit culture and work characteristics of 235 nursing department staff in 13 units as a precursor to changing their care delivery model. Nursing-unit culture was measured by means of the Nursing Unit Cultural Assessment Tool (NUCAT-2) (Coeling and Simms, 1993). Performance was measured in terms of unit skill mix, cost, worked hours per patient day, quality assurance, documentation of care planning and discharge, and patient satisfaction. The premature report of this study prevents any conclusions from being drawn. Only one unit had reached its one-year evaluation stage, and the reported results suggest a thinly veiled cost-cutting exercise.

A rigorous study by Shortell *et al.* (2000) assessed the impact of TQM and organisational culture on performance in terms of a wide range of outcomes for 3045 CABG patients. Culture was measured by means of the competing values framework (Quinn and Rohrbaugh, 1981; Cameron and Freeman, 1991; Gillies *et al.*, 1992). Performance was measured in terms of risk-adjusted clinical outcomes, functional health status, patient satisfaction and cost.

The results showed that although a two- to fourfold difference in all major clinical CABG care endpoints was observed among the 16 hospitals, little of this variation was associated with TQM or organisational culture. Patients who received CABG from hospitals with high TQM scores were more satisfied with their nursing care ($P = 0.005$) but were more likely to have lengths of stay exceeding 10 days ($P = 0.0003$). A supportive group culture was associated with shorter postoperative intubation times ($P = 0.01$) but longer operating-room times ($P = 0.004$). A supportive group culture was also associated with higher patient physical ($P = 0.005$) and mental ($P = 0.01$) functional health status scores six months after CABG.

Zimmerman *et al.* (1993) also failed to find evidence for a link between culture and performance in a study involving 3672 ICU admissions, 316 nurses and 202 physicians in nine ICUs. Culture was assessed using a combination of interviews, direct observations and questionnaires, including the Organisational Culture Inventory (Cooke and Lafferty, 1987). Effectiveness was measured by the ratio of actual/predicted hospital death rate, and efficiency was measured by the ratio of actual/predicted length of ICU stay.

On the basis of each unit's risk-adjusted mortality rates, nine out of 42 ICUs were selected for intensive on-site analysis by investigators who were blinded to the actual mortality rates. Using semi-structured interviews, examination of physical artefacts and observation, each investigator developed a summary report which was shared and discussed by study members, and was then combined with all summary reports to create a composite report for each unit. In this way a listing of the 'best' and 'worst' cultures, leadership, co-ordination, communication and problem-solving practices was developed, together with the potential effect on ICU performance. Each investigator also rated the nine ICUs (from best to worst) according to their anticipated final risk-adjusted mortality ranking.

The results of the on-site assessments indicated that superior organisational practices among the ICUs were related to a patient-centred culture, strong medical and nursing leadership, effective communication and co-ordination, and open, collaborative approaches to solving problems and managing conflict. However, the on-site case studies failed to identify accurately units with significantly better or worse performance in terms of risk-adjusted survival.

This failure may be due to a lack of mismatch between the subjectively based on-site investigations and the objective assessment of actual risk-adjusted mortality. Interestingly, Zimmerman *et al.* (1993) concluded that the cause of the problem lay in their performance criteria. For example, Unit A performed well in terms of risk-adjusted mortality rate, but less well in terms of length of ICU stay. In contrast, Unit H displayed superior efficiency with regard to length of ICU stay, but had a poor risk-adjusted mortality ratio:

> We believe the inaccuracy of the rankings was related to an inability to distinguish these measures (e.g. effectiveness vs. efficiency) and the absence of an objective value-free process for arriving at criteria on which to evaluate performance.
>
> (Zimmerman *et al.*, 1993, p. 1450)

The final healthcare organisational study of culture and performance, by Zimmerman *et al.* (1994), is a follow-up of their earlier study (Zimmerman *et al.*, 1993). The later study focuses on two ICUs with marked differences in risk-adjusted survival. Objective measures of ICU performance were compared with subjective assessments by unit staff members and the research team. The actual hospital death rate was 20.7% for Unit 1 and 6.25% for Unit 2. When compared with the 42 ICUs in the APACHE III study, the ratio of actual to mean predicted mortality at Unit 1 (1.21) was significantly worse, and at Unit 2 (0.76) it was significantly better. The mean ICU length of stay was 5.2 days for Unit 1 and 4 days for Unit 2. The ratio of mean actual to mean predicted ICU length of stay for Unit 2 (0.89) was significantly better than that for Unit 1 (0.93), and not significantly different from the mean value for all 42 study units. The ratios of mean actual to mean predicted ICU resource use for Units 1 and 2 were significantly worse than those for the 42 APACHE III study units. The mortality data identify the two study units as Units H and B from the 1993 study. The findings of the 1994 study do not differ from those of the 1993 study. Neither the global judgements of the on-site investigators nor the self-evaluation by unit physicians and nurses accurately ranked Units 1 and 2 according to risk-adjusted mortality. In addition, on-site observations and questionnaire data regarding culture, leadership, co-ordination, communication and problem solving/conflict management did not clearly distinguish between high- and low-performing units.

The findings of Zimmerman *et al.* (1993) and Shortell *et al.* (2000) do little to resolve the question of the relationship between culture and performance. However, they do help to highlight a paradox at the heart of performance assessment in healthcare, which may also explain why the link with organisational culture, if it exists, is so difficult to determine. There is as little consensus about defining performance as there is about defining culture. Although it is frequently presented as a hard-nosed, bottom-line concept, performance is almost as nebulous, elusive and complex as culture. Consider its two basic contents, namely effectiveness and efficiency. The relationship between mortality and length of ICU stay is not simple. A patient who is moved from the ICU too early might relapse and return to the ICU, the two stays possibly costing more in terms of health and money than one longer stay. Even a longer stay in a step-down unit or ward will bump up the cost. And that principle of shunting the problem further down the line, and not measuring the full consequences, appears to be typical of much healthcare performance assessment. A growing body of research suggests that setting performance criteria can be dysfunctional by actually creating additional costs, disbenefits and other distortions, by focusing undue effort on symptoms (e.g. waiting-lists) instead of addressing causes (Smith, 1995). Shorter ICU stays could also increase morbidity and may cause death. If shorter ICU stays can contribute to increased cost and mortality/morbidity, then length of ICU stay on its own is not a reliable measure of efficiency. Risk-adjusted mortality on its own is an equally blunt instrument. At the very least it should be used together with morbidity, which is of course more difficult both to define and to measure. The likelihood is that measures such as length of ICU stay and death rates are selected for use as performance criteria because they are convenient – days and bodies are easy to count. Zimmerman *et al.* (1994) are therefore correct to raise the issue of adequate measurement. Once we accept that performance is a fundamentally contested domain, the difficulty of reconciling culture and performance through such simplistic equations as 'strong culture = superior performance' begin to appear surreally naive.

# Discussion

## Summary of results

Of 18 studies included in this review, nine tended to support a link between organisational culture and performance. Nine studies were performed in non-healthcare organisations and nine were performed in healthcare organisations. Of the nine non-healthcare settings, five studies found some evidence of a link between organisational culture and performance – one ideographic study (Frame *et al.*, 1989) and four nomothetic studies (Denison, 1984; Cameron and Freeman, 1991; Kotter and Heskett, 1992; Banerjee, 1995). Of four other studies that did not support the hypothesis, three found no convincing positive evidence for such a link (Rousseau, 1990; Quick, 1992; Fairfield-Sonn, 1993) and one (Lewis, 1994) presented positive evidence against a link. Of the nine healthcare studies, four supported a link between organisational culture and performance – one ideographic study (Jackson, 1997) and three nomothetic studies (Argote, 1989; Gerowitz *et al.*, 1996; Gerowitz, 1998). Of the five healthcare studies that did not support the hypothesis (Nystrom, 1993; Zimmerman *et al.*, 1993, 1994; Rizzo *et al.*, 1994; Shortell *et al.*, 2000), none found evidence against the link.

# Methodological issues

Partly due to the methodological diversity of the studies included in this review no formal comparative assessment of methodological quality was undertaken. Methods ranged from overt non-participant observation to telephone and face-to-face interviews, and the study of artefacts and behaviour, archived data, financial performance data and questionnaires. A number of studies triangulated data from different methodologies. Most of the studies were cross-sectional, and would have benefited from a longitudinal approach with data collection over several time-points. In the case of interventions designed to alter organisational culture and performance, a 'before-and-after' approach is preferable, but was used in only a minority of the non-healthcare studies (Kotter and Heskett, 1992; Lewis, 1994) and in none of the healthcare studies. Although it is difficult to draw firm conclusions from such a diverse sample of studies, there was no discernible connection between the level of methodological rigour and whether or not the studies supported a link between organisational culture and performance.

# Aspects of culture assessed

Most of the studies included in this review focused on culture level 1a (patterns of behaviour) (Schein, 1985; Ott, 1989) and level 2 (attitudes, beliefs and values) (Schein, 1985). Five studies (Cameron and Freeman, 1991; Banerjee, 1995; Gerowitz *et al.*, 1996; Gerowitz, 1998; Shortell *et al.*, 2000) used the competing values framework to measure attitudes, beliefs and values. Of these five studies, only one (Shortell *et al.*, 2000) did not find evidence of a link between organisational culture type and performance. Of three studies that examined culture level 1 (artefacts), Frame *et al.* (1989) analysed mission statements, Quick (1992) examined artefacts created by the founder/leader, and Zimmerman *et al.* (1994) observed awards and ceremonies. All three studies found these artefacts to be informative and significant relative to performance (although we were not persuaded of this by Quick). None of the studies examined level 3 (underlying assumptions).

Most investigators acknowledge Schein's analysis (Schein, 1985) of organisational culture into the following three levels of ascending importance: 1, artefacts; 2, beliefs and values; 3, unspoken assumptions. Schein maintains that the essence of an organisation's culture lies in its unspoken assumptions. These assumptions may be conceived as an organisational unconscious, of which artefacts and values are conscious manifestations. However one views the psychoanalytical metaphor, it is generally acknowledged that organisational cultures are like icebergs in that only the peak is visible above the surface. According to Schein (1985), the basic technique for examining the submerged culture is to look for discrepancies between espoused values and actual practices (artefacts). By exploring these faults in the fabric of organisational life, Schein asserts, it is possible to bring an underlying pattern of assumptions to the surface. If we accept Schein's model, and as none of the included studies attempted this depth and rigour of analysis, it should not be surprising that a relationship between culture and performance has proved elusive.

Failure to engage unspoken cultural assumptions could lead to apparently random effects of culture on performance. However, these effects can be brought to order by reinterpreting the relationship in terms of cultural assumptions and performance. Thus in one non-healthcare study (Frame *et al.*, 1989), culture change and performance improvement arose from a crisis that was triggered by the destruction of cultural assumptions, which must have occurred when almost the entire workforce was replaced by a new, inexperienced workforce. In another study (Banerjee, 1995), an *assumption* of client centredness is a stronger explanation for superior service outcomes than an espoused value of client centredness. Kotter and Heskett (1992) found that firms which showed consistently good performance over time tended to possess *core* values that emphasised the importance of an adaptive culture. Core values sound closer to unspoken assumptions than to espoused beliefs, and present a more convincing motivation.

Turning to the healthcare studies, Jackson (1997) found that a relationship existed between the outpatient department's culture and patients' attendance, but that its precise nature remained unclear. In a deeply entrenched culture like that of the NHS, a systematic failure by staff to attend to patients promptly, and a fear (among patients) of contacting the hospital in order to change an appointment are probably only explicable in terms of unspoken assumptions informing relationships. Espoused values would only have a similar effect if personnel were coerced to obey them, or if behaviour patterns were disconnected from assumptions, both of which are unlikely. Argote (1989) found that agreement about norms *between* groups is positively and significantly associated with the effectiveness of emergency units, whereas the relationship between effectiveness and normative agreement *within* units is weaker and less clear. This could indicate that between-group norms were measured at a deeper and therefore more consistent level than the within-group norms – that deeper level being closer to assumptions than to normative beliefs.

In Part 2 we discussed the choice between assessing organisational culture types (e.g. the competing values framework) and continuous variables (e.g. the OCI). The way in which organisational culture is assessed is perhaps less important than the aim of the assessment. As no definitive assessment of something as complex as an organisation's culture is likely to be possible, the assessment should be used as a means of opening a dialogue within and across organisational boundaries. By an iterative process of diagnosis and dialogue, organisational participants may become conscious of the basic assumptions that silently control their thoughts and actions, and they may even revise them in more constructive directions.

However, there are potential dangers to this process. Individuals might learn surprising and even distressing facts about themselves – that they have been blind to their own motivations or manipulated to ends and by means that they may decry. Learning is a constructive process as well as a reconstructive one. In making sense of the past, we use a narrative about the past to inform the present and the future. Thus, learning about NHS culture is also a making of NHS culture. When we say 'NHS culture is introspective and hierarchical' (Gerowitz et al., 1996), we define some possibilities but we also deny others. Paradoxically, assertion involves an acknowledgement that the opposite is also true. Nowhere is this more apposite than in the culture of a vast organisation such as the NHS, which penetrates every corner of our society, is interwoven with national culture, and is composed of a variety of different subcultures. Whether each subculture is a variation on an overarching theme, or whether the whole culture is a laminate of semi-autonomous occupational identities, it would be difficult to decide. However, it is likely that for each assertion about NHS culture we will find a contradiction embodied in another part or person.

# Appropriateness of outcomes

The studies included in this review examined a variety of different outcomes, raising the question of how to define performance and which performance-related outcomes are appropriate for assessing an organisation's culture. As there is no consensus on which outcomes are affected by culture, we should not be surprised that many studies fail to find any effect. A related issue concerns the degree of real separation between the independent and dependent variables in some of the included studies. It is questionable, for example, to assess the effect of values on employee loyalty and commitment (Gerowitz et al., 1996), which are values in themselves. Might it be more accurate to view those

'outcomes' as being embedded in the culture? Similarly, can subjective judgements by managers of their organisation's performance be viewed as being
external to the organisation's culture type (Gerowitz, 1998)? There is a danger
of confusing cause and effect, and thus confounding assessment.

Few investigators have sought to measure outcomes external to culture.
Shortell *et al.* (2000) examined a range of CABG outcomes, while Zimmerman
*et al.* (1993) assessed ICU mortality and length of stay. Although a two- to
fourfold difference in all major clinical CABG care endpoints was observed
by Shortell *et al.* (2000) among the 16 hospitals, little of this variation was
associated with TQM or organisational culture. Zimmerman *et al.* (1993) failed
to identify accurately units with significantly better or worse performance
in terms of risk-adjusted survival. Both sets of authors explain their results in
terms of the highly complex and interdependent processes of healthcare provision. Although valid, this adds little to what we already know, and it will not
diminish the demand for measurable improvements in the quality of healthcare.

Culture and culture change interventions fall into the category of *diffuse*
health technologies (Keen *et al.*, 1995; Scott, 1996, 1997). Diffuse health technologies intervene systemically rather than topically. Their emphasis is on
changing organisational processes that contribute to service delivery, not
impacting directly on providers' behaviour. Thus the chain of causality linking
diffuse health technologies with service outcomes tends to be multiple, discon-
tinuous and difficult to trace. Diffuse technologies are a necessary complement
to structural organisational changes. Without a diffuse technological component, structural alterations are likely to lead to anachronistic attitudes and
behaviour in novel settings. However, revised attitudes and behaviour may be
slow to yield tangible results because a process of sedimentation has to occur,
whereby patient centredness, for example, gradually becomes an unspoken
premise upon which the entire sociotechnical paraphernalia of care delivery is
grounded. Therefore the corollary of this review, based upon all three parts
(dealing with the theory of organisational culture, organisational culture
assessment tools and organisational culture and performance, respectively), is
that we should conceptualise the relationship between organisational culture
and performance differently. Organisational culture is like a lotus plant. The
lotus flower sits on the surface of the water in full view, but the plant is rooted
firmly in the mud. If we imagine unspoken cultural assumptions as a rhizome,
hidden in the rich silt of the organisational unconscious, out of sight or
conscious mind, if we think of beliefs and values as the stems rising from those
roots to the surface, and of artefacts and behaviour as the leaves and flowers, we
can begin to see where cultural intervention of a radical kind needs to be
directed. The only way to remove, replace or transplant the culture lotus is by
handling the roots, thereby involving the whole plant. In order to do that one
has to immerse oneself in the water — the ecological substrate — which in this
analogy represents the organisational environment or ecology. What is the

connection between this botanical analogy and performance? Does the lotus flower serve a double role as both the expression of culture *and* its performance outcomes? Or is it more apposite to view artefacts and performance outcomes as different, interdependent genera in an organisational ecology? The former captures something of the paradoxical relationship between culture and performance – the way in which they sometimes appear to be different, and at other times the same, alternatively subordinate to each other. The latter captures a more satisfying view of the relationship as part of organisational 'pond life', culture and performance being at once actors and contextual factors in a shared ecosystem. However we view the leaves and flowers (artefacts and behaviour), and however hard we peer into the water in order to examine the stems (values) that disappear into the murky depths, the hypothesis is the same. In order to truly understand an organisation's culture, we need to gain access to its roots – those deep and unspoken assumptions upon which the rest of the plant depends. This is a different and perhaps more challenging task than collecting observations or questionnaire responses, and so far as connecting the enquiry to performance outcomes is concerned, it remains a largely unexplored avenue of research.

A theme introduced by cognitive approaches to culture change is the role of organisational learning. Argyris and Schon (1978) developed the concept of the learning organisation in terms of single-loop vs. double-loop feedback. The notion of double-loop feedback or learning transforms the limited cybernetic concept of feedback (e.g. in which a missile guidance system constantly corrects the weapon's trajectory by reference to the changing position of the target, or a surgeon guides an endoscope by reference to the images that it sends back to a monitor) into a more advanced concept (in which an intelligent remote guidance system would learn to improve its ability from each individual launch, or the surgeon would learn to develop endoscopic technology, not just his or her own skills, on the basis of each operation, by accident, creative reflection, experimentation, communicating with technical developers, dissemination, etc.).

The success of clinical governance may well depend on this distinction between mere feedback and learning – upon a distinction between governance as direct feedback between strategy and performance, and governance as an oblique intervention whereby policy and strategy evolve in response to their own strengths and weaknesses as revealed in practice. In general, the performance indicator systems used by the NHS to date have signally failed to evolve in this way, and learning does not seem to have occurred.

Developing NHS organisational culture implies learning about learning. Recent research in the USA has made some headway in this direction (Ferlie and Shortell, 2001). For example, a group-oriented culture that emphasises affiliation, teamwork, co-ordination and participation appears to be associated with greater implementation of continuous quality improvement practices (Shortell *et al.*, 1995). There is also some evidence that a patient-centred culture that incorporates aligned compensation incentives is positively associated with the implementation of clinical guidelines (Shortell *et al.*, 2001). By contrast, a hierarchical culture that emphasises rules, regulations and formal reporting relationships appears to be negatively associated with the implementation of quality improvement (Ferlie and Shortell, 2001).

The research programme headed by Shortell at Berkeley involves a hybrid style of investigation combining some of the characteristics of the qualitative organisational case study with the quantitative elements of biomedical research. Further methodological developments are needed in order to investigate organisational culture and performance in the NHS, both because culture is not an operational term and cannot therefore be subjected to classical scientific investigation, and because the insights generated are characteristically double-loop in nature. Organisational research investigates the social, political, economic and technical processes that occur within the organisation. Only by gaining an understanding of such processes can we begin to make sense of the relationship between organisational structure, culture and performance.

# Conclusion

Is there a link between organisational culture and performance? What is the nature of that relationship? How can we intervene in the NHS to change culture and affect performance? The empirical studies reviewed in this part of the book do not provide clear answers to any of these questions. We would have been surprised if they had because, in effect, answers would have been suddenly provided to some of the key underlying questions asked about organisations since at least the 1930s – questions concerning organisational forms, human motivation, the meaning of work, leadership and management, and so on. Not so much questions as perennial themes of organisational research.

What we do find depends on our interpretation of an apparently inconsistent pattern of results. We have tried to make sense of this by highlighting what has been clearly missed, or at least avoided, by investigators, namely the level of unspoken cultural assumptions. Discovering assumptions is likely to be more intensive and to involve more interpretation than assessing values. It may be found that there is less variation in shared basic assumptions between organisational members and between subcultures, with the result that intensive effort at the level of assumptions will be more productive than more expansive efforts at 'higher' levels. However, we do not propose to substitute one level for others, for two reasons. First, in order to generate a representation of a culture, we need to investigate all three levels and their interdependency. Secondly, according to Schein's model (Schein, 1985), it is only through dialogue about artefacts, behaviour and values that underlying assumptions can be approached. By analogy, access to the organisational unconscious is negotiated through manifest symbols, effects, cognitions and behaviour. Tracing the labyrinthine connections between latent and manifest organisational culture promises to be a fascinating and difficult undertaking.

There is another interpretation. According to the post-Freudian, post-Marxist, post-Hegelian, post-modernist spirit of the current era, everything happens at the surface of things. Everything is fleeting, playful and superficial. The familiar relationship between latent and manifest phenomena, which underpins the social and psychological structures and dynamics discussed by Marx and Freud, is revealed as purely ideological — or, as Paul Valéry discovered, *what is most deep is the skin* (Deleuze, 1990). If that is true, a project to diagnose underlying culture and its effects on outcomes would be misguided, and any examination of deeper structures and processes risks becoming a metaphysical flight of fancy. All we can say about this critique is that meaning is as meaning does — if we believe a thing to be real, then it is real enough to affect and even to dominate our thoughts, emotions and actions. If the superficial configuration of organisational culture and performance yields only a faint pattern, as appears to be the case on the basis of the studies reviewed here, perhaps this is because that is all there is. Perhaps the intuition that what we term an organisation's culture *must* affect its outcomes is no more than a trace of an old-fashioned notion of a surface-depth topology of organisational and social existence. There are at least two reasons for reserving judgement on this point. The first is that, notwithstanding the more or less rigorous investigations of academic researchers, an entire industry has been built on the idea that organisational culture and performance are indeed linked. We therefore need to know whether this industry is built on sand or solid rock, and whether to spend scarce public money on organisational developmental programmes based on that rationale. Secondly, the whole story about organisational culture and performance is a long way from being told. There have been few empirical studies, and most of them are methodologically weak. The potential cost of giving up the search at this relatively early stage is greater than the cost of taking it forward along a path, which both methodologically and thematically seems to be relatively clear.

We have considered the thematic dimension in terms of incorporating the level of assumptions into future investigations. The methodological dimension is more problematic. This is not the stage at which to revisit the qualitative/quantitative debate. We have already signalled the need for a clinical approach to analysing cultural assumptions according to a protocol suggested by Schein (1985). Our final comment is reserved for a more general protocol for the evaluation of diffuse health technologies. With focal technologies (e.g. a drug or surgical technique), the assessment is rightly made in terms of patient outcomes and cost. Because diffuse technologies (e.g. culture change) are intended to have systemic effects, their direct contribution to patient outcomes may not be traceable. Thus methods of measuring the effectiveness of process interventions are required, although this is excluded by at least one authority (St Leger *et al.*, 1992). An alternative approach is to set assessment criteria that are congruent with process interventions. For instance, if a system of digital data exchange between hospital departments is intended to improve communication and reduce the volume of circulating paperwork, then an assessment should begin by examining those effects. It does not make sense to assess such an intervention directly in terms of patient outcomes, since these are contingent upon interventions that are focused on the point of care. With a culture change intervention, such as an attempt to inculcate different values, the immediate assessment would be of value change. Value change in turn can be assessed in terms of behavioural change (and vice versa), and behaviour change can be assessed in terms of patient outcomes. It is illogical to short-circuit the assessment logic by jumping straight from culture or culture change to patient outcomes. Not only does it neglect to scrutinise links in the intervening causal chain, which is important for understanding how the intervention works or is inhibited from working, but it is also contradictory to at once recognise the importance of culture by intervening at a specific level, and only then to treat it as the 'black box' mediating between input and output.

However, the evaluative framework of Keen *et al.* (1995), which is designed to guide the evaluation of diffuse technologies, may be useful for guiding those intent on assessing culture in terms of performance outcomes. Of particular value is the advocacy of whole-organisation studies, site-specific studies and patient-focused studies as part of the same assessment:

> Whether the focus of evaluation is a particular service within the hospital (4b) or a patient group (4c), the strategy is to break down the domain into constituent elements and conduct studies focusing on specific detailed questions. The sum of the answers to the right questions should yield good data to inform judgements about the technology as a whole.
>
> (Keen *et al.*, 1995, p. 159)

By adhering to this loose framework and by including cultural assumptions along with artefacts, behaviour and values in the evaluation, a more comprehensive and sensitive approach to the study of organisational culture may be possible in the short term. In the longer term, we suspect and hope that a number of hitherto unknown methodologies, unimagined by conventional health services research, await discovery.

# References

- Ackroyd S and Crowdry P (1991) Can culture be managed? Working with 'raw' material: the case of the English slaughterhouse. *Personnel Rev.* **19**: 3–11.
- Alexander M (1978) Organizational norms oppinionnaire. In: J Pfeiffer and J Jones (eds) *The 1978 Annual Handbook for Group Facilitators*. University Associates, La Jolla, CA.
- Allaire Y and Firsirotu M (1984) Theories of organizational culture. *Organiz Stud.* **5**: 193–226.
- Alpander G (1990) Relationship between commitment to hospital goals and job satisfaction: a case study of a nursing department. *Health Care Manag Rev.* **15**: 51–62.
- Alvesson M (1992) Leadership as social integrative action: a study of a computer consultancy company. *Organiz Stud.* **13**: 185–209.
- Andrews J and Hirsch P (1983) Ambushes, shootouts and knights of the round table: the language of corporate takeovers. In: L Pondy, P Frost, G Morgan and T Dandridge (eds) *Organizational Symbolism*. JAI, Greenwich, CT.
- Argote L (1989) Agreement about norms and work-unit effectiveness: evidence from the field. *Basic Appl Soc Psychol.* **10**: 131–40.
- Argyris C and Schon D (1978) *Organizational Learning*. Addison-Wesley, Reading, MA.
- Arnold H and Feldman D (1982) A multivariate analysis of the determinants of job turnover. *J Appl Psychol.* **67**: 350–60.
- Banerjee M (1995) Desired service outcomes: toward attaining an elusive goal. *Admin Soc Work.* **19**: 33–53.
- Barnard C (1938) *The Functions of the Executive*. Harvard University Press, Cambridge, MA.
- Bass B (1985) *Leadership and Performance Beyond Expectations*. Free Press, New York.
- Bass B and Alviolo B (1990) The implications of transactional and transformational leadership for individual, team and organizational development. *Res Organiz Change Dev.* **4**: 231–72.
- Bass B and Alviolo B (1993) Transformational leadership: a response to critiques. In: M Chemers and R Ayman (eds) *Leadership Theory and Research: perspectives and directions*. Academic Press, New York.
- Bate P (1984) The impact of organizational culture on approaches to organizational problem solving. *Organiz Stud.* **5**: 43–66.
- Bateson G (1941) Experiments in thinking about ethnographic observed material. *Phil Sci.* **8**.

- Bennis W and Nanus B (1985) *Leaders: the strategies for taking charge.* Harper & Row, New York.
- Beyer J and Trice H (1988) The communication of power relations in organizations through cultural rites. In: M Jones, M Moore and R Sayder (eds) *Inside Organizations: understanding the human dimension.* Sage, Newbury Park, CA, pp. 141–57.
- Boje D, Fedor D *et al.* (1982) Myth making: a qualitative step in OD interventions. *J Appl Behav Sci.* **18**: 17–28.
- Bougon M (1983) Uncovering cognitive maps. In: G Morgan (ed.) *Beyond Method.* Sage, Beverly Hills, CA, pp. 173–88.
- Brown A (1995) *Organisational Culture.* Pitman, London.
- Brown J (1954) *The Social Psychology of Industry.* Penguin, Harmondsworth.
- Brown JAC (1963) *Techniques of Persuasion. Pelican Original.* Penguin, Harmondsworth.
- Bryman A (1996) Leadership in organizations. In: S Clegg, C Hardy and W Nord (eds) *Handbook of Organization Studies.* Sage, London, pp. 277–92.
- Buckingham M and Coffman C (2000) *First Break All the Rules.* Simon and Schuster, London.
- Burns J (1978) *Leadership.* Harper & Row, New York.
- Burns T and Stalker G (1961) *The Management of Innovation.* Tavistock, London.
- Burrell G (1996) Normal science, paradigms, metaphors, discourses and genealogies of analysis. In: S Clegg, C Hardy and W Nord (eds) *Handbook of Organization Studies.* Sage, London, pp. 642–58.
- Burrell G and Morgan G (1979) *Sociological Paradigms and Organisational Analysis.* Gower, Aldershot.
- Calas MB and Smircich L (1996) From 'the woman's' point of view: feminist approaches to organization studies. In: S Clegg, C Hardy and W Nord (eds) *Handbook of Organization Studies.* Sage, London, pp. 218–57.
- Cameron KS (1978) Measuring organizational effectiveness in institutions of higher education. *Admin Sci Quart.* **23**: 482–95.
- Cameron KS (1981) Domains of organizational effectiveness in colleges and universities. *Acad Manag J.* **24**: 25–47.
- Cameron KS (1986) A study of organizational effectiveness and its predictors. *Manag Sci.* **32**: 86–112.
- Cameron K and Freeman S (1991) Culture, congruence, strength and type: relationship to effectiveness. *Res Organiz Change Dev.* **5**: 23–58.
- Campbell J (1977) On the nature of organizational effectiveness. In: P Goodman and J Pennings (eds) *New Perspectives on Organizational Effectiveness.* Jossey-Bass, San Francisco, CA.
- Clarke B (1970) *The Distinctive College: Antioch, Reed and Swarthmore.* Aldine, Chicago.
- Coeling H and Simms L (1993) Facilitating innovation at the nursing unit level through cultural assessment. Part 1. How to keep management ideas from falling on deaf ears. *J Nurs Admin.* **23**: 46–53.
- Conger J (1989) *The Charismatic Leader: behind the mystique of exceptional leadership.* Jossey-Bass, San Francisco, CA.

- Cooke R and Lafferty J (1987) *Organizational Culture Inventory (OCI)*. Human Synergistics, Plymouth, MI.
- Cooke R and Rousseau D (1988) Behavioural norms and expectations: a quantitative approach to the assessment of organizational culture. *Group Organiz Stud.* **13**: 245–73.
- Cooke T and Campbell D (1979) *Quasi-Experimentation: design and analysis issues for field settings*. Rand McNally, Chicago, IL.
- Cooley C (1909) *Social Organization*. Scribner, New York.
- Corzine JB (1997) Machiavellianism and management: a review of single-nation studies exclusive of the USA and cross-national studies. *Psychol Rep.* **80**: 291–304.
- Davies B, Philp A *et al.* (1993) *CCQ Manual and User's Guide*. Saville and Holdsworth Ltd, Thames Ditton.
- De Bivort L (1985) Fast-tracking the transformation of organizations. In: J Adams (ed.) *Transforming Work*. Miles River Press, Alexandria, VA, pp. 243–52.
- Deal T and Kennedy A (1982) *Corporate Cultures*. Addison-Wesley, Reading, MA.
- Deleuze G (1990) *The Logic of Sense*. Columbia University Press, New York.
- Deleuze G and Guattari F (1983) *Anti-Oedipus*. Athlone, London.
- Denison D (1984) Bringing corporate culture to the bottom line. *Organiz Dynamics.* **13**: 5–22.
- Douglas MT and Isherwood BC (1979/1996) *The World of Goods: towards an anthropology of consumption*. Routledge, London.
- Durkheim E (1958). In: AW Gouldner (ed.) *Socialism and Saint-Simon*. Antioch, Yellow Springs, OH.
- Dyer W (1985) The cycle of cultural evolution in organizations. In: R Kilmann, M Saxton, R Serpa *et al.* (eds) *Gaining Control of the Corporate Culture*. Jossey-Bass, San Francisco, CA, pp. 200–29.
- Emmerson J (1973) Behaviour in private places: sustaining definitions of reality in gynaecological examinations. In: G Salaman and K Thompson (eds) *People and Organisations*. Longman, Harlow, pp. 358–71.
- England G and Keaveny T (1969) The relationship of managerial values and administrative behaviour. *Manpower Appl Psychol.* **3**: 63–75.
- Everett J, Stening B *et al.* (1982) Some evidence for an international managerial culture. *J Manag Stud.* **19**: 153–62.
- Fairfield-Sonn J (1993) Moving beyond vision: fostering cultural change in a bureaucracy. *J Organiz Change Manag.* **6**: 43–55.
- Ferlie E and Shortell SM (2001) Improving the quality of health care in the United Kingdom and the United States: a framework for change. *Milbank Q.* **79**: 281–315.
- Fiedler F (1967) *A Theory of Leadership Effectiveness*. McGraw-Hill, New York.
- Fiedler F (1993) The leadership situation and the black box in contingency theories. In: M Chemers and R Ayman (eds) *Leadership Theory and Research: perspectives and directions*. Academic Press, New York.
- Fiedler F and Garcia J (1987) *Improving Leadership Effectiveness: cognitive resources and organizational performance*. John Wiley & Sons, New York.

- Fletcher B and Jones F (1992) Measuring organizational culture: the cultural audit. *Manag Audit J.* **7**: 30–6.
- Fox A (1985) *Man Mismanagement.* Hutchinson, London.
- Fox N (1993) *Postmodernism, Sociology and Health.* Open University Press, Buckingham.
- Frame R, Nielsen W *et al.* (1989) Creating excellence out of crisis: organizational transformation at the *Chicago Tribune. J Appl Behav Sci.* **25**: 109–22.
- French W and Bell C (1978) *Organizational Development.* Prentice-Hall, Englewood Cliffs, NJ.
- Gagliardi P (1986) The creation and change of organizational cultures: a conceptual framework. *Organiz Stud.* **7**: 117–34.
- Geertz C (1973) *The Interpretation of Cultures.* Basic Books, New York.
- Georgopoulos B (1965) Normative structure variables and organizational behavior. *Hum Relations.* **18**: 155–69.
- Gerowitz MB (1998) Do TQM interventions change management culture? Findings and implications. *Qual Manag Health Care.* **6**: 1–11.
- Gerowitz M, Lemieux-Charles L *et al.* (1996) Top management culture and performance in Canadian, UK and US hospitals. *Health Serv Manag Res.* **6**: 69–78.
- Gibb C (1947) The principles and traits of leadership. *J Abnorm Soc Psychol.* **42**: 267–84.
- Gillies R *et al.* (1992) *Culture Survey.* Health Policy and Management School of Public Health, Berkeley, CA.
- Gioia D and Chittipeddi K (1991) Sensemaking and sensegiving in strategic change initiation. *Strategic Manag J.* **12**: 433–48.
- Goffman E (1959) *The Presentation of Self in Everyday Life.* Doubleday, Garden City, NY.
- Goodenough W (1971) *Culture, Language and Society.* Addison-Wesley, Reading, MA.
- Goodridge D and Hack B (1996) Assessing the congruence of nursing models with organizational culture: a quality improvement perspective. *J Nurs Care Qual.* **10**: 41–8.
- Gouldner A (1959) Organizational analysis. In: RK Merton *et al.* (eds) *Sociology Today: problems and prospects.* Basic Books, New York.
- Greene C (1975) The reciprocal nature of influence between leader and subordinate. *J Appl Psychol.* **60**: 187–93.
- Hackman J and Oldham G (1975) Development of the Job Diagnostic Survey. *J Appl Psychol.* **60**: 159–70.
- Haire M, Ghiselli E *et al.* (1966) *Managerial Thinking: an international study.* John Wiley & Sons, New York.
- Handy C (1995) *Gods of Management: the changing work of organizations.* Oxford University Press, Oxford.
- Harris L and Cronen V (1979) A rules-based model for the analysis and evaluation of organizational communication. *Commun Q.* **27**: 12–28.
- Harrison R (1972) Understanding your organization's character. *Harvard Bus Rev.* **5**: 119–28.

- Harrison R (1975) Diagnosing organization ideology. In: J Jones and J Pfeiffer (eds) *The 1975 Annual Handbook for Group Facilitators*. University Associates, La Jolla, CA, pp. 101–7.
- Hatch M (1993) The dynamics of organizational culture. *Acad Manag Rev.* **18**: 657–93.
- Heisenberg W (1958) *Physics and Philosophy*. Harper Brothers, New York.
- Hofstede G (1980) *Culture's Consequences: international differences in work-related values*. Sage, Beverly Hills, CA.
- Hofstede G and Bond MH (1988) The Confucius connection: from cultural roots to economic growth. *Organiz Dynamics.* **16**: 4–21.
- Hofstede G, Neuijen B *et al.* (1990) Measuring organizational cultures: a qualitative and quantitative study across 20 cases. *Admin Sci Q.* **35**: 286–316.
- Homans G (1950) *The Human Group*. Harcourt Brace, New York.
- House R (1977) A 1976 theory of charismatic leadership. In: J Hunt and L Larson (eds) *Leadership: the cutting edge*. Southern Illinois University Press, Carbondale, IL.
- Ingersoll GL, Kirsch JC *et al.* (2000) Relationship of organizational culture and readiness for change to employee commitment to the organization. *J Nurs Admin.* **30**: 11–20.
- Isabella L (1990) Evolving interpretations as a change unfolds: how managers construe key organizational events. *Acad Manag J.* **33**: 7–41.
- Jackson S (1997) Does organizational culture affect outpatient DNA rates? *Health Manpower Manag.* **23**: 233–6.
- Jacques E (1952) *The Changing Culture of a Factory*. Dryden, New York.
- Jaynes J (1976) *The Origin of Consciousness in the Breakdown of the Bicameral Mind*. Houghton Mifflin, Boston, MA.
- Jenkins W (1947) A review of leadership studies with particular reference to military problems. *Psychol Bull.* **44**: 54–77.
- Jones J and Pfeiffer J (1975) *The 1975 Annual Handbook for Group Facilitators*. University Associates, La Jolla, CA.
- Jones W (1961) *The Romantic Syndrome: toward a new method in cultural anthropology and the history of ideas*. Martinus Wijhaff, The Hague.
- Jung C (1923) *Psychological Types*. Routledge & Kegan Paul, London.
- Jung C (1973) *Four Archetypes: mother/rebirth/spirit/trickster*. Princeton University Press, Princeton, NJ.
- Katzenbach J and Smith D (1993) *The Wisdom of Teams: creating the high-performance organization*. Harvard Business School, Boston, MA.
- Keen J, Bryan S *et al.* (1995) Evaluation of diffuse technologies: the case of digital imaging networks. *Health Policy.* **34**: 153–66.
- Kennedy I (2001) *Learning from Bristol: Public Inquiry into Children's Heart Surgery at the Bristol Royal Infirmary 1984–1995*. The Stationery Office, London.
- Kennedy J (1982) Middle LPC leaders and the contingency model of leadership effectiveness. *Organiz Behav Hum Perform.* **31**: 1–14.

- Kilmann R (1984) *Beyond the Quick Fix: managing five tracks to organizational success.* Jossey-Bass, San Francisco, CA.
- Kilmann R and Saxton M (1983) *Kilmann-Saxton Culture Gap Survey.* Organizational Design Consultants, Inc., Pittsburgh, PA.
- Koch S and Deetz S (1981) Metaphor analysis of social reality in organizations. *J Appl Commun Res.* **9**: 1–15.
- Korman A (1966) 'Consideration', 'initiating structure' and organizational criteria – a review. *Pers Psychol.* **19**: 349–61.
- Kotter J (1990) *A Force for Change: how leadership differs from management.* Free Press, New York.
- Kotter J and Heskett J (1992) *Corporate Culture and Performance.* Macmillan, New York.
- Krackhardt D and Stern R (1988) Informal networks and organizational crises: an experimental simulation. *Soc Psychol Q.* **51**: 123–40.
- Kuhn T (1970) *The Structure of Scientific Revolutions.* University of Chicago Press, Chicago, IL.
- Lackoff G and Johnson M (1980) *Metaphors We Live By.* University of Chicago Press, Chicago, IL.
- Lafferty J (1973) *Level I: Life Styles Inventory self-description.* Human Synergistics, Plymouth, MI.
- Lawrence P and Lorsch J (1967) *Organization and Environment.* Harvard University Press, Cambridge, MA.
- Lawrence P and Dyer D (1983) *Renewing American Industry.* Free Press, New York.
- Lewin K (1952) *Field Theory in Social Science.* Tavistock, London.
- Lewis D (1994) Organizational change: relationship between reactions, behaviour and organizational performance. *J Organiz Change Manag.* **7**: 41–55.
- Lim B (1995) Examining the organizational culture and organizational performance link. *Leadership Organiz Dev J.* **16**: 16–21.
- Linstead S and Grafton-Small R (1992) On reading organizational culture. *Organiz Stud.* **13**: 331–55.
- Lisney B and Allen C (1993) Taking a snapshot of cultural change. *Personnel Manag.* **February**: 38–41.
- Litwinenko A and Cooper CL (1994) The impact of trust status on corporate culture. *J Manag Med.* **8**: 8–17.
- Lord R and Maher K (1991) *Leadership and Information Processing: linking perceptions and performance.* Unwin Hyman, Cambridge, MA.
- Louis M (1980) Organizations as culture-bearing milieux. In: L Pondy, P Frost, G Morgan and T Dandridge (eds) *Organizational Symbolism.* JAI, Greenwich, CT, pp. 39–54.
- Lowin A and Craig C (1968) The influence of performance on managerial style: an experimental object lesson in the ambiguity of correlational data. *Organiz Behav Hum Perform.* **3**: 440–58.

- Lundberg C (1985) On the feasibility of cultural intervention. In: P Frost, L Moore, M Louis, C Lundberg and J Martin (eds) *Reframing Organizational Culture*. Sage, Newbury Park, CA, pp. 169–85.
- Lyotard JF (1984) *The Postmodern Condition: a report on knowledge*. Manchester University Press, Manchester.
- McDaniel C (1995) Organizational and ethics work satisfaction. *J Nurs Admin*. **25**: 15–21.
- McDaniel C and Stumpf L (1993) The organizational culture: implications for nursing service. *J Nurs Admin*. **23**: 54–60.
- Mackenzie S (1995) Surveying the organizational culture in an NHS trust. *J Manag Med*. **9**: 69–77.
- Machiavelli N (1992) *The Prince*. WW Norton, New York.
- McNulty T and Ferlie E (2002) *Re-Engineering Health Care: the complexities of organizational transformation*. Oxford University Press, Oxford.
- Mann R (1959) A review of the relationship between personality and performance in small groups. *Psychol Bull*. **56**: 241–70.
- Manz C and Sims H (1991) SuperLeadership: beyond the myth of heroic leadership. *Organiz Dynamics*. **19**: 18–35.
- Marris P (1986) *Loss and Change*. Routledge & Kegan Paul, London.
- Martin J (1992) *Cultures in Organizations: three perspectives*. Oxford University Press, New York.
- Martin J and Powers M (1983) Truth of corporate propaganda: the value of a good war story. In: L Pondy, P Frost, G Morgan and T Dandridge (eds) *Organizational Symbolism*. JAI, Greenwich, CT.
- Martin J and Seihl C (1983) Organizational culture and counterculture: an uneasy symbiosis. *Organiz Dynamics*. **12**: 52–64.
- Mason C (1992) Non-attendance at out-patients clinics: a case study. *J Adv Nurs*. **17**: 554–60.
- Meek L (1988) Organizational culture: origins and weaknesses. *Organiz Stud*. **9**: 453–73.
- Meyer A (1981) How ideologies supplant formal structures and shape responses to environments. *J Manag Stud*. **19**: 45–61.
- Michaels C and Spector P (1982) Causes of employee turnover: a test of the Mobley, Griffeth, Hand and Meglino model. *J Appl Psychol*. **67**: 53–9.
- Miles RH and Cameron KS (1982) *Coffin Nails and Corporate Strategy*. Prentice-Hall, Englewood Cliffs, NJ.
- Miles R and Snow C (1978) *Organizational Strategy, Structure and Process*. McGraw-Hill, New York.
- Mintzberg H (1979) *The Structuring of Organizations*. Prentice-Hall, Englewood Cliffs, NJ.
- Mitroff I (1982) *Stakeholders of the Mind*. Academy of Management Meetings, New York City.

- Mitroff I (1983) *Stakeholders of the Organizational Mind.* Jossey-Bass, San Francisco, CA.
- Mitroff I and Kilmann R (1976) On organizational stories: an approach to the design and analysis of organizations through myths and stories. In: R Kilmann, L Pondy and D Slevin (eds) *The Management of Organization Design.* Elsevier, New York.
- Moday R, Steers R *et al.* (1979) The measurement of organizational commitment. *J Voc Behav.* **14**: 224–47.
- Morgan G (1980) Paradigms, metaphors and puzzle solving in organization theory. *Admin Sci Q.* **25**: 605–22.
- Morgan G (1986) *Images of Organisation.* Sage, Beverly Hills, CA.
- Morgan G and Smircich L (1980) The case for qualitative research. *Acad Manag Rev.* **5**: 491–500.
- Morgan G, Frost P *et al.* (1983) Organizational symbolism. In: L Pondy, P Frost, G Morgan and T Dandridge (eds) *Organizational Symbolism.* JAI, Greenwich, CT.
- Neuman E (1955) *The Great Mother: an analysis of archetype.* Princeton University Press, Princeton, NJ.
- Neuman E (1970) *The Origins and History of Consciousness.* Princeton University Press, Princeton, NJ.
- Nossiter V and Biberman G (1990) Projective drawings and metaphor: an analysis of organizational culture. *J Manag Psychol.* **5**: 13–16.
- Nutt PC (1976) Models for decision making in organizations. *Acad Management Rev.* **2**: 84–98.
- Nystrom PC (1993) Organizational cultures, strategies and commitments in health care organizations. *Health Care Manag Rev.* **18**: 43–9.
- Ott J (1989) *The Organizational Culture Perspective.* Dorsey, Chicago, IL.
- Ouchi W and Wilkins A (1985) Organizational culture. *Ann Rev Sociol.* **11**: 457–83.
- Ouchi WG (1981) *Theory Z.* Addison-Wesley, Reading, MA.
- Parker M (2000) *Organizational Culture and Identity.* Sage, London.
- Pascale R and Athos A (1981) *The Art of Japanese Management.* Simon & Schuster, New York.
- Pasmore W (1988) *Designing Effective Organizations: the sociotechnical systems perspective.* John Wiley & Sons, New York.
- Pearce J, Robbins D *et al.* (1987) The impact of grand strategy and planning formality on financial performance. *Strateg Manag J.* **8**: 125–34.
- Peters T (1978) Symbols, patterns and settings: an optimistic case for getting things done. *Organiz Dynamics.* **7**: 3–23.
- Peters T and Waterman R (1982) *In Search of Excellence.* Harper & Row, New York.
- Pettigrew A (1979) On studying organizational culture. *Admin Sci Q.* **24**: 570–81.
- Pfeffer J (1981) Management as symbolic action: the creation and maintenance of organizational paradigms. In: L Cummings and B Staw (eds) *Research in Organizational Behavior.* JAI, Greenwich, CT.
- Podsakoff P, Todor W *et al.* (1984) Situational moderators of leader reward and punishment behaviors: fact or fiction. *Organiz Behav Hum Perform.* **34**: 21–63.

- Pondy L and Mitroff I (1979) Beyond open system models of organization. In: L Cummings and B Staw (eds) *Research in Organizational Behavior*. JAI, Greenwich, CT.
- Porter L, Steers R *et al.* (1974) Organizational commitment, job satisfaction, and turnover among psychiatric technicians. *J Appl Psychol.* **59**: 603–9.
- Quick J (1992) Crafting an organizational culture: Herb's hand at Southwest Airlines. *Organiz Dynamics.* **21**: 45–56.
- Quinn J (1978) Strategic change, logical incrementalism. *Sloan Manag Rev.* **20**: 7–21.
- Quinn R (1988) *Beyond Rational Management: mastering the paradoxes and competing demands of high performance*. Jossey-Bass, San Francisco, CA.
- Quinn R and Rohrbaugh J (1981) A competing values approach to organizational effectiveness. *Public Product Rev.* **5**: 122–40.
- Quinn R and McGrath M (1984) The transformation of organizational cultures: a competing values perspective. In: P Frost, M Louis, C Lundberg, L Moore and J Martin (eds) *Organizational Culture*. Sage, Beverly Hills, CA.
- Reilly N and Orsak C (1991) A career stage analysis of career and organizational commitment in nursing. *J Vocat Behav.* **39**: 311–30.
- Ritzer G (1975) *Sociology: a multi-paradigm science*. Allyn and Bacon, Boston, MA.
- Rizzo JA, Gilman MP *et al.* (1994) Facilitating care delivery: redesign using measures of unit culture and work characteristics. *J Nurs Admin.* **24**: 32–7.
- Roethlisberger F and Dickson W (1939) *Management and the Worker*. Harvard University Press, Cambridge, MA.
- Rossi I and O'Higgins E (1980) The development of theories of culture. In: I Rossi (ed.) *People in Culture*. Praeger, New York.
- Rousseau D (1990) Normative beliefs in fund-raising organizations. *Group Organiz Stud.* **13**: 448–60.
- Rusbult C and Farrell D (1983) A longitudinal test of the investment model: the impact on job satisfaction, job commitment, and turnover of variations in rewards, costs, alternatives and investments. *J Appl Psychol.* **68**: 429–38.
- Rush M, Thomas J *et al.* (1977) Implicit leadership theory: a potential threat to the internal validity of leader behavior questionnaires. *Organiz Behav Hum Perform.* **20**: 93–110.
- St Leger A, Schnieden H *et al.* (1992) *Evaluating Health Services Effectiveness*. Open University Press, Buckingham.
- Sashkin M (1988) The visionary leader. In: J Conger and R Kanungo (eds) *Charismatic Leadership: the elusive factor in organizational effectiveness*. Jossey-Bass, San Francisco, CA.
- Sathe V (1983) Implications of a corporate culture: a manager's guide to action. *Organiz Dynamics.* **12**: 4–23.
- Schein E (1964) The mechanism of change. In: W Bennis *et al.* (eds) *Interpersonal Dynamics*. Dorsey Press, Homewood, IL.
- Schein E (1985) *Organizational Culture and Leadership*. Jossey-Bass, San Francisco, CA.
- Schein E (1990) Organizational culture. *Am Psychol.* **45**: 109–19.

- Schein E (1999) *The Corporate Culture Survival Guide.* Jossey-Bass, San Franscisco, CA.
- Scott J (1996) Work and organisation. In: *Management Systems and Sciences.* University of Hull, Hull.
- Scott J (1997) *The Nature and Evaluation of Diffuse Health Technologies.* Warwick Business School Research Bureau, Warwick.
- Seago J (1995) *Work Group Culture, Workplace Stress and Hostility: correlations with absenteeism and turnover in hospital nurses.* University of California, San Francisco, CA.
- Seago J (1996) Work group culture, stress and hostility: correlations with organizational outcomes. *J Nurs Admin.* **26**: 39–47.
- Seago J (1997) Organizational culture in hospitals: issues in measurement. *J Nurs Meas.* **5**: 165–78.
- Selznick P (1957) *Leadership in Administration: a sociological interpretation.* Harper & Row, New York.
- Shortell SM, Zimmerman J *et al.* (1994) The performance of intensive-care units: does good management make a difference? *Med Care.* **32**: 508–25.
- Shortell SM, O'Brien J *et al.* (1995) Assessing the impact of continuous quality improvement/total quality management: concept versus implementation. *Health Serv Res.* **30**: 377–401.
- Shortell SM, Jones RH *et al.* (2000) Assessing the impact of total quality management and organizational culture on multiple outcomes of care for coronary artery bypass graft surgery patients. *Med Care.* **38**: 207–17.
- Shortell SM *et al.* (2001) Implementing evidence-based medicine: the role of market pressures, compensation incentives and culture in physician organizations. *Med Care.* **39**(7): Suppl. 1–79–1–91.
- Siehl C and Martin J (1981) *Learning Organizational Culture.* Working paper. Stanford University, Stanford, CA.
- Siehl C and Martin J (1984) The role of symbolic management: how can managers effectively transmit organizational culture? In: J Hunt, D Hosking, C Schriesheim and R Stewart (eds) *Leaders and Managers: international perspectives on managerial behavior and leadership.* Pergamon, New York.
- Sieveking N, Bellet W *et al.* (1993) Employees' views of their work experience in private hospitals. *Health Serv Manag Res.* **6**: 129–38.
- Sims H and Lorenzi P (1992) *The New Leadership Paradigm.* Sage, Newbury Park, CA.
- Singh R (1998) Redefining psychological contracts with the US workforce: a critical task for strategic human resources planners in the 1990s. *Hum Resource Manag.* **37**: 61–9.
- Smircich L (1983) Concepts of culture and organizational analysis. *Admin Sci Q.* **28**: 339–58.
- Smircich L and Morgan G (1982) Leadership: the management of meaning. *J Appl Behav Sci.* **18**: 257–73.
- Smith A (1970) *The Wealth of Nations.* Penguin, Harmondsworth.
- Smith P (1995) On the unintended consequences of publishing performance data in the public sector. *Int J Pub Admin.* **18**: 277–310.

- Sprott W (1958) *Human Groups*. Penguin, Harmondsworth.
- Stevenson K (2000) Are your practices resistant to changing their clinical culture? *Prim Care Rep.* **2**: 19–20.
- Stogdill R (1948) Personal factors associated with leadership: a survey of the literature. *J Psychol.* **25**: 35–71.
- Stogdill R (1950) Leadership, membership and organization. *Psychol Bull.* **47**: 1–14.
- Stogdill R (1974) *Handbook of Leadership: a survey of theory and research*. Free Press, New York.
- Thomas C, Ward M *et al.* (1990) Measuring and interpreting organizational culture. *J Nurs Admin.* **20**: 17–24.
- Tichy N (1982) Managing change strategically: the technical, political and cultural keys. *Organiz Dynamics.* **Autumn**: 59–80.
- Tichy N and Devanna M (1986) *The Transformational Leader*. John Wiley & Sons, New York.
- Tierney W (1987) The semiotic aspects of leadership: an ethnographic perspective. *Am J Semiotics.* **5**: 233–50.
- Tierney W (1989) Symbolism and presidential perceptions of leadership. *Rev Higher Educ.* **12**: 153–66.
- Trice H and Beyer J (1984) Studying organizational cultures through rites and ceremonials. *Acad Manag Rev.* **9**: 653–69.
- Trice H and Beyer J (1990) Cultural leadership in organizations. *Organiz Sci.* **2**: 149–69.
- Trice H and Beyer J (1993) *The Cultures of Work Organizations*. Prentice-Hall, Englewood Cliffs, NJ.
- Trist E and Bamforth K (1951) Some social and psychological consequences of the longwall method of coal getting. *Hum Relations.* **4**: 3–38.
- Turner S (1977) Complex organizations as savage tribes. *J Theory Soc Behav.* **7**: 99–125.
- Turner S (1983) Studying organization through Levi-Strauss's structuralism. In: G Morgan (ed.) *Beyond Method*. Sage, Beverly Hills, CA.
- Van de Ven A and Astley W (1981) Mapping the field to create a dynamic perspective on organization design and behavior. In: A Van de Ven and W Joyce (eds) *Perspectives on Organization Design and Behavior*. John Wiley & Sons, New York.
- Van Maanen J (1973) Observations on the making of policemen. *Hum Organiz.* **32**: 407–18.
- Wacker G (1981) Toward a cognitive methodology of organizational assessment. *J Appl Behav Sci.* **17**: 114–29.
- Weick KE (1976) Educational organizations as loosely coupled systems. *Admin Sci Quart.* **21**: 1–19.
- Weick K (1979a) Cognitive processes in organizations. In: L Cummings and B Staw (eds) *Research in Organizational Behavior*. JAI, Greenwich, CT.
- Weick K (1979b) *The Social Psychology of Organizing*. Addison-Wesley, Reading, MA.

- Westley F and Mintzberg H (1989) Visionary leadership and strategic management. *Strateg Manag J.* **10**: 17–32.
- Wilkins A and Martin J (1980) *Organizational Legends.* Working paper. Stanford University, Stanford, CA.
- Wilkins AL and Ouchi WG (1983) Efficient cultures: exploring the relationship between culture and organizational performance. *Admin Sci Quart.* **28**: 468–81.
- Yiannis G (1999) Organizational culture. In: G Yiannis (ed.) *Organizations in Depth.* Sage, London.
- Zaleznik A (1977) Managers and leaders: are they different? *Harvard Bus Rev.* **55**: 67–78.
- Zimmerman J, Knaus W *et al.* (1991) Organizational correlates with ICU efficiency and effectiveness. *Crit Care Med.* **19**: 35.
- Zimmerman J *et al.* (1993) Improving intensive care. Observations based on organizational case studies in nine intensive-care units: a prospective, multicentre study. *Crit Care Med.* **21**: 1443–51.
- Zimmerman J *et al.* (1994) Intensive care at two teaching hospitals: an organizational case study. *Am J Crit Care.* **3**: 129–38.

# Index